COLOR TASTE TE...

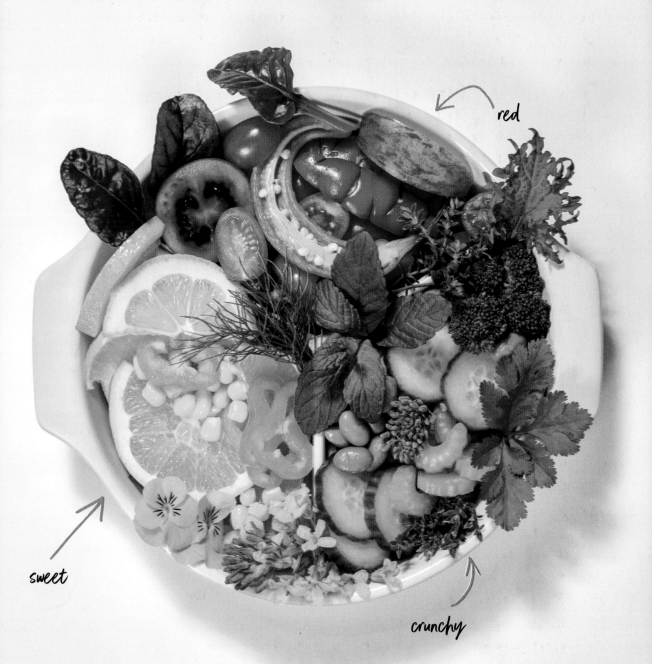

red

sweet

crunchy

COLOR

TASTE

TEXTURE

Recipes for Picky Eaters, Those with Food Aversion, and Anyone Who's Ever Cringed at Food

MATTHEW BROBERG-MOFFITT

AVERY ⟪ AN IMPRINT OF PENGUIN RANDOM HOUSE ⟪ NEW YORK

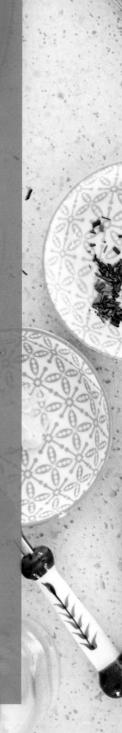

AVERY

an imprint of Penguin Random House LLC
penguinrandomhouse.com

Most Avery books are available at special quantity discounts for bulk purchase for sales promotions, premiums, fund-raising, and educational needs. Special books or book excerpts also can be created to fit specific needs. For details, write SpecialMarkets@penguinrandomhouse.com.

Library of Congress Cataloging-in-Publication Data

Names: Broberg-Moffitt, Matthew, author.
Title: Color taste texture: recipes for picky eaters, those with food aversion, and anyone who's ever cringed at food / Matthew Broberg-Moffitt.
Description: New York: Avery, an imprint of Penguin Random House, [2023] | Includes index.
Identifiers: LCCN 2022049759 (print) | LCCN 2022049760 (ebook) | ISBN 9780593538593 (trade paperback) | ISBN 9780593538609 (epub)
Subjects: LCSH: Cooking. | Food preferences. | Taste buds. | LCGFT: Cookbooks.
Classification: LCC TX714.B762 2023 (print) | LCC TX714 (ebook) | DDC 641.5—dc23/eng/20221122
LC record available at https://lccn.loc.gov/2022049759
LC ebook record available at https://lccn.loc.gov/2022049760

Printed in the United States of America

10 9 8 7 6 5 4 3 2 1

BOOK DESIGN BY LORIE PAGNOZZI

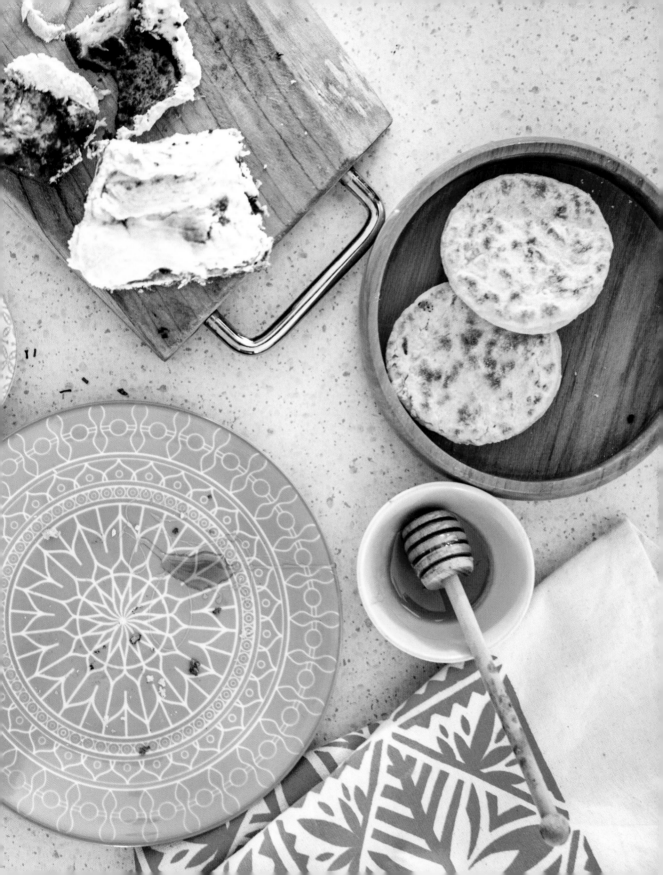

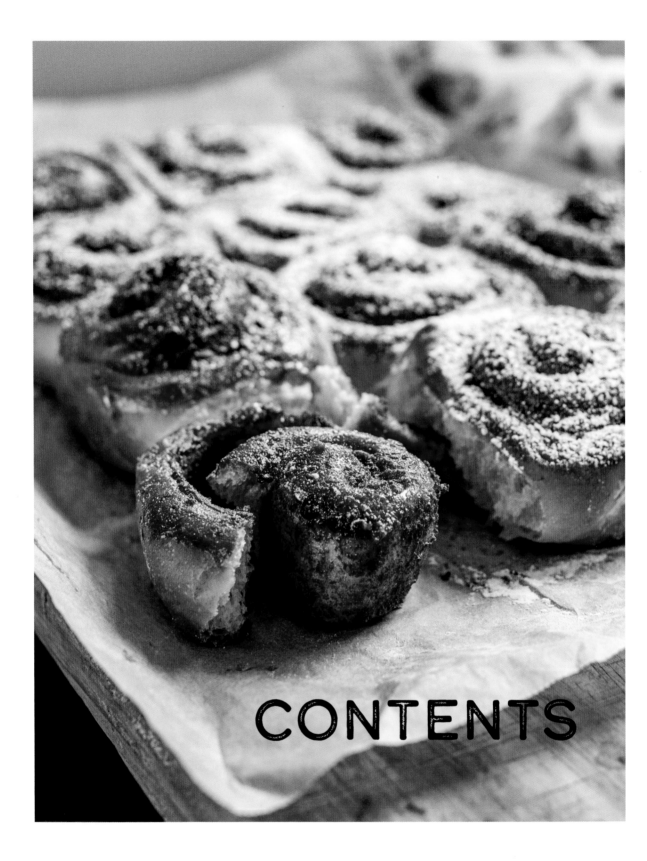

CONTENTS

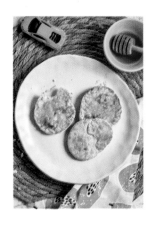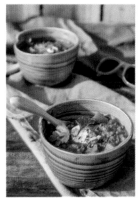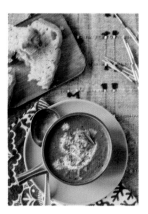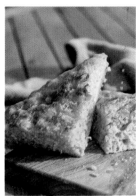

CHAPTER 8—RECIPES

BREAKFAST

LUNCHTIME

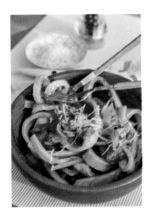
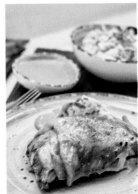
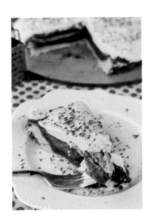
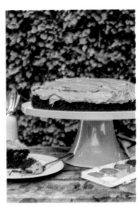

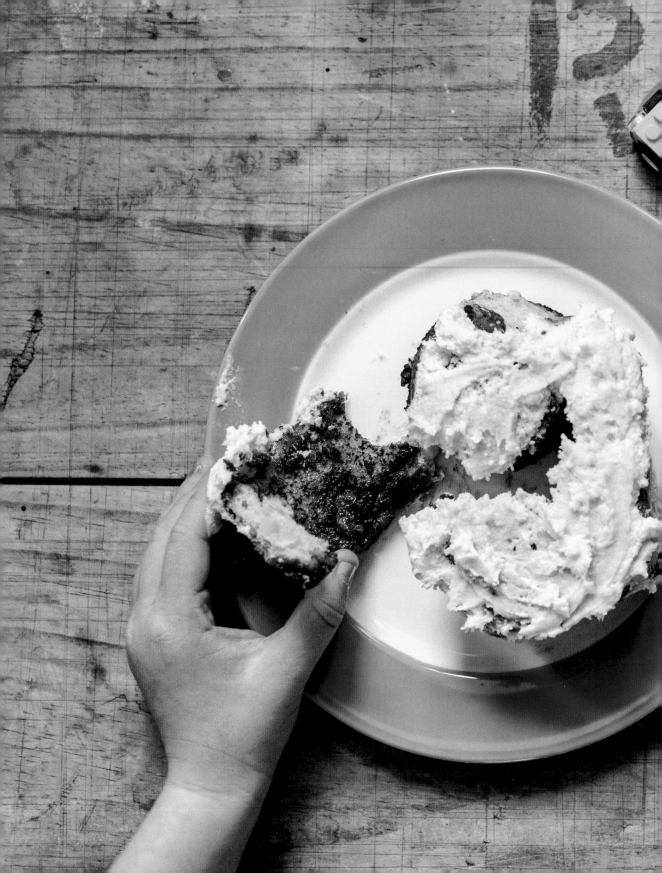

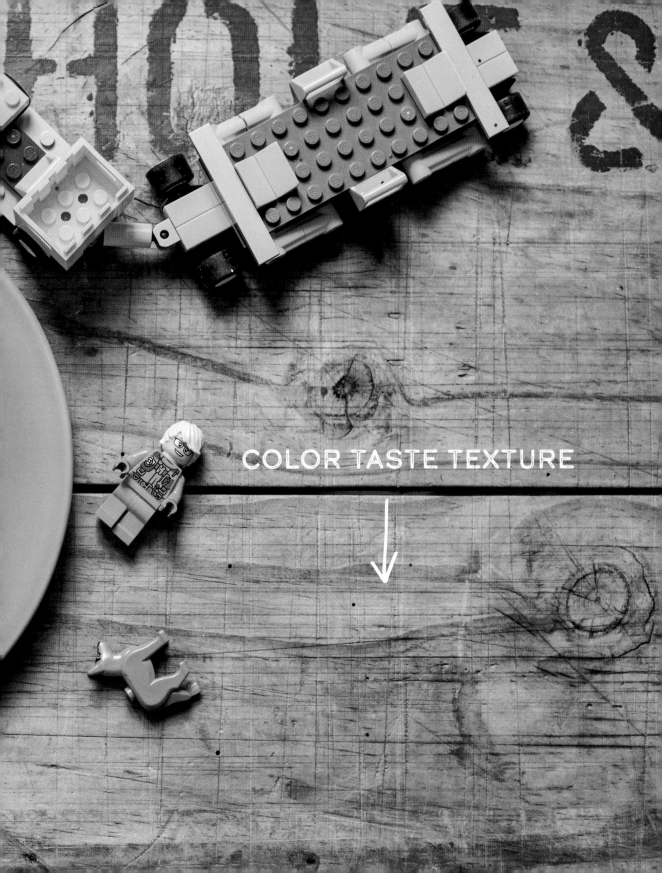

COLOR TASTE TEXTURE

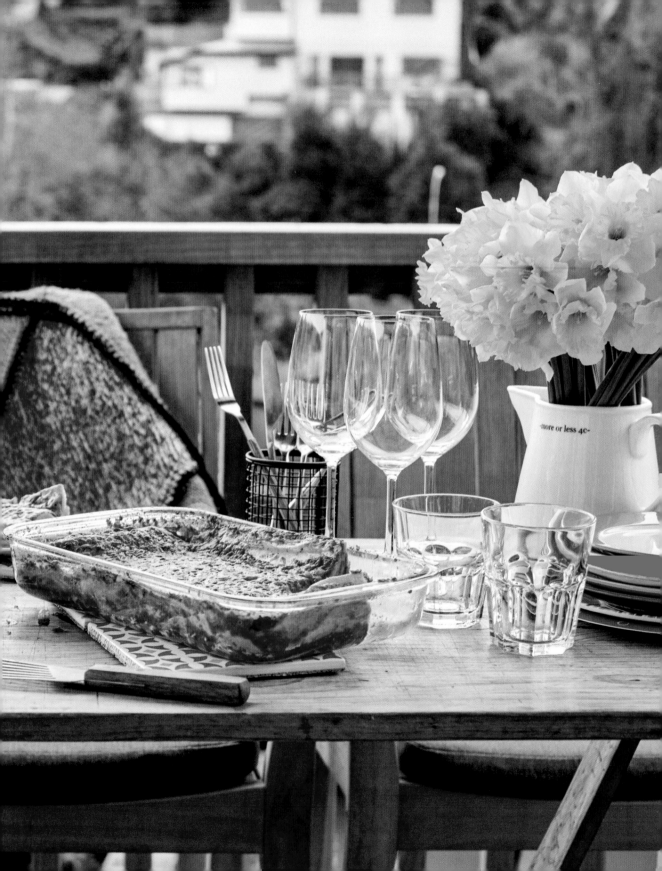

CHAPTER 1

COLOR TASTE TEXTURE

ME? WHY ME?

"Can I get that plain? No sauce, condiments, vegetation, or foliage?"

If you've ever uttered those words, this might be the cookbook for you. My name is Matthew Broberg-Moffitt, and I'm autistic and food averse. I'm also a classically trained chef. Now, that may sound counterintuitive, and in fact it is. I'm a classically trained chef who has never worked in the food industry because some food is just gross.

I don't mean "gross" as a value statement toward the food itself, or toward the people who eat the stuff I don't. Having aversions has been a part of my life for as long as I can remember. There have been changes over the years with some foods entering the "safe list" in a slow, almost glacial, manner. I have a son, who also has food aversions. His are different from my own, and sometimes I must take a step back and say, "It's okay that he doesn't like watermelon. He doesn't like strawberries, or most berries. It's okay." Likewise, your aversions will not be judged. This is a safe place! Even if I don't share your preference, it will be honored and respected.

Perhaps most important, this cookbook isn't going to try to sneak in food that you absolutely don't want to eat. Instead, it's all about working within your parameters or those of the food-averse person you're cooking for. For example, if your kid or loved one doesn't like the taste or smell of onions, then stop putting onions in their food—but if they don't like the *texture* of onions, we can work with that. I will show you how to prepare onions so that their texture is palatable. If your kid only eats chicken fingers and mashed potatoes and absolutely refuses anything else, make them *the best* chicken fingers and mashed potatoes. If they are getting adequate nutrition and calories, this cookbook isn't going to try to force anything else on them.

I can't tell you how many times I sat at a kitchen table as a child, long after everyone else had finished, and a well-meaning adult wouldn't let me leave until I cleaned my plate. It was always a deeply embarrassing and uncomfortable experience. I've always liked to follow rules, and to consistently disappoint adults when it came to food was traumatic. I wasn't diagnosed with autism until I was an adult, and while I'd like to think that it would have made a difference, in this instance I believe the results would have been the same. After all, there wasn't much by way of acceptance of food aversion. There still isn't! The market and internet advice space are replete with ways to "trick" picky eaters instead. It's my hope that radical, enthusiastic acceptance of food aversion will help reframe these experiences and change social attitudes in a positive and meaningful way. If one kid can have a less traumatic childhood because of this, I'll be a truly happy camper.

GLOSSARY

There are a lot of terms that get bandied about in cooking, and it can sometimes be easy for me to forget that not everyone knows them. It doesn't help that they are frequently not in English, and even when they are in seeming "layperson's" tongue, they aren't always self-explanatory. To help facilitate your understanding I've created a glossary.

Dice—To cut into quarter-inch cubes using a sharp kitchen knife.

Mince—To cut into an even smaller size than to dice.

Crush—To smoosh, aggressively, often with the back of a knife on a cutting board.

Sweat—To cook over low heat, often an aromatic, so that the moisture is released. The final product will often be translucent and slightly crunchy.

Steam—To heat indirectly utilizing a moist medium. When cooking aromatics in a pan, where the heat is low and the pan is overcrowded, you often steam as a result, as the sweat produced by the cooking of the vegetables then evaporates and cooks the aromatics beside them. Steaming varies from sweating, in that the end product is more homogeneous in texture and softer in consistency.

Caramelize—To produce a Maillard reaction, wherein the surface of the food turns a darker brown and the released moisture and carbohydrates become sweeter as they are condensed.

Brown—Similar to caramelization, but with a much less dramatic effect.

Chiffonade—To slice things like herbs into long, thin ribbons, facilitated by rolling the subject in question.

Roux—To produce this backbone of sauces and the tangzhong bread method (see page 14), a small amount of flour is cooked on the stove in a saucepan in either water or, more commonly, butter (especially in the French Mother Sauces).

Mirepoix—A French culinary aromatic tradition of cooking diced onion, celery, and carrot in butter.

Soffritto—An Italian culinary aromatic tradition of cooking diced onion, celery, and carrot in olive oil (and sometimes also with butter!).

Aromatics—Things like vegetables and herbs that are heated in fat or oil in the beginning of the dish to provide flavor.

Carryover—A phenomenon where foods retain heat and continue to cook even when removed from the heating element.

Leavener—Something that helps produce lift and rise to things like breads and custards—examples include yeast, baking soda, baking powder, and eggs.

The Five Mother Sauces—Foundational elements to numerous dishes in French culinary tradition. They include béchamel, a butter and flour roux–thickened cream base; tomato, a tomato base; hollandaise, an egg yolk and lemon juice base; espagnole, a reduced brown sauce; and velouté, made from butter, flour, and clear stock.

Low and Slow—A popular cooking method for large pieces of inexpensive, tougher cuts of meat, such as a brisket or shoulder. These pieces have a few things in common, such as being particularly fatty or fibrous, due to the place on the animal they come from. By preparing these foods at a low cooking temperature, over longer times, we can help break down what might otherwise be a very difficult texture and make it much more comparable to more expensive, leaner cuts of meat. Alternatively, a very tender and lean cut of beef might be able to be sliced very thin and cooked purely in acids in a shockingly rapid amount of time, due to the difference in how the fibers and muscles are developed where it's derived.

FOOD AVERSION IN A NUT-FREE NUTSHELL

While it would be easy to assume that you are familiar with food aversion and that's why you picked up this cookbook, even those who experience it haven't necessarily given it much consideration. So let's start with a simple thought experiment.

> You may be saying to yourself, "A thought experiment in a cookbook?!" Yes: *Color Taste Texture*'s approach to food aversion is as much a philosophy as it is a tool kit and guide. If someone can identify and empathize, it's much easier to normalize.

Remember back to your childhood. Were there any foods that you just thought were completely yuck? If the answer is yes, take a brief inventory of what it was about that food that you hated—and possibly continue to hate—so much.

Maybe you can't explain why; it's just nasty. Simple enough. Now dig a little deeper: Was it the taste? Was it *only* the taste? Was there something about the texture that turned your stomach? Perhaps the color reminded you of something that shouldn't be consumed. It might have made you physically sick when you ate it, even without a diagnosed allergen or sensitivity.

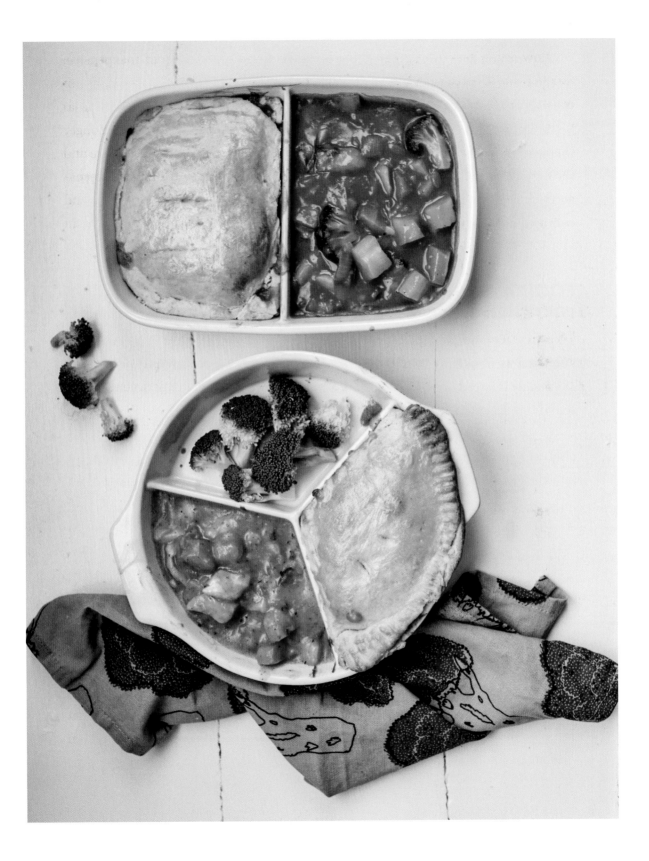

If you don't have an example, imagine you're going out to eat and spot [blank] on the menu. What food makes you say, "I don't like [blank]?" Would you eat it if it were on your plate?

Most of us have *something* that would qualify as a food aversion. So let's enter this journey with this core thought: Food aversion is okay. It's not something I'm trying to cure. It's not my intention to force change. My mission is to encourage acceptance of food aversion, remove the stress around the dinner table, and make eating as much of a joyful and enjoyable experience as possible.

FOOD AVERSIONS AND FIXATIONS: SAME COIN, DIFFERENT SIDES

There are food-averse folks who can verbalize quite clearly what they won't eat, and I just as frequently hear about those who will *only* eat a specific thing. This is commonly referred to as a *samefood*. It's important to recognize that these two presentations are often intertwined.

If you only eat smooth soup, it is easy to avoid anything that's crunchy. If you only eat a specific brand of frozen breaded chicken nuggets, you find comfort in the knowledge that what you are going to eat is both familiar and unproblematic.

NUTRITION AND SAMEFOODS

Ever since I announced that I was writing a cookbook, I've been asked questions by parents and partners of the food averse about getting their loved ones to eat more than just their favored samefoods. This is a triage situation: See to their critical and fundamental needs first. How?

My first question to these seekers is: Are the food averse getting adequate nutrition every day? If the answer is yes, I encourage them to take both a deep breath and a step back. If their people are eating enough calories, protein, and fiber ("enough" meaning that their digestive system is basically regular), it's much better to take a more relaxed approach. Accept that your loved one has a samefood. Do your best to be supportive of their choices and provide opportunities for them to explore safely and without judgment.

If the answer is no, it's time to find creative nutrition solutions that work within their palette (or palate!) and preferences. That might be with a prepackaged nutrition supplement or with a more holistic and tailored option (such as Gavin's Vanilla Shake, page 71). Above all, I don't want people to starve or suffer.

AUTISM AND OTHER ASSOCIATED CONDITIONS

Food aversion is a well-known comorbid condition with autism spectrum disorders. However, it isn't unique to autism and not all autistics experience it.

Some additional common conditions associated with food aversion:

- Avoidant restrictive food intake disorder is an eating disorder that features food aversion without body dysmorphia.

- Nearly everyone is familiar with the food cravings and adverse food reactions of pregnancy, as the senses are enhanced (especially smell, which is a critical factor in taste).

- Chronic migraines and their associated enhanced sense of smell are known to induce temporary food aversions, in addition to nausea.

- Motion sickness can make eating a chore, and exposure to specific foods may trigger nausea.

- Previous food poisoning can create a fierce averse response when something reminds you of that experience.

This is not an exhaustive list, but hopefully it gives a little glimpse into the complexity of food aversion. It might also help to illustrate that the food averse are often responding to heightened sensitivity. Autistics and other neurodiverse individuals with difficulty blocking out stimuli would logically experience an increased incidence of food aversion as a result.

FOOD PREFERENCES PROFILE AND WORKSHEET

Wouldn't life be easier if everyone had a list of foods that they especially liked and didn't like? While it doesn't guarantee that Grandma or Grandpa is going to honor your children's wishes (or your own, for that matter), it does give the food averse some feeling of autonomy and agency when they know that their personal preferences are being listened to and respected. The Nonspeaking Feedback sheet can be a reference for nonspeaking folk, so they can either point to an area on the page that is problematic or write out an answer on a separate piece of paper. Ask the individual what they don't like or do like about the food in question and follow their guidance.

Before we move forward, take a minute to fill out this Food Preferences Profile Worksheet—for yourself or with your loved one—to produce a list of safe foods and the big no-go foods for easy reference.

FOOD PREFERENCES PROFILE WORKSHEET

NAME:

AGE:

FOOD ALLERGIES OR SENSITIVITIES:

DIETARY NEEDS:

NO-GO FOODS:

SAMEFOODS:

SAFE VEGGIES:

SAFE SNACKS:

NONSPEAKING FEEDBACK

COLOR

TASTE

TEXTURE

SMELL

PLATING

ENVIRONMENT

DON'T FEEL WELL (NOT THE FOOD)

I would also recommend taking some time to establish some expectations with your family as you move forward on the path of acceptance. Because food aversion and neurodiversity go together like peanut butter and chocolate (unless one or the other—or both—is a food aversion), encouraging change may require an explicit set of stated and visually listed guidelines about food and eating that everyone in the family abides by.

Your family may find that the example below requires amendment or alteration for your unique needs, and that is okay. The key tenet is one of unconditional, enthusiastic acceptance. With that spirit in mind, feel free to tweak as needed. This is just a template.

If possible, you may also find that a meal schedule posted ahead for the week helps establish a sense of security or safety—but only attempt it if you can be reasonably certain that you are able to follow the schedule, as sudden changes may lead to additional difficulties.

GUIDELINES ABOUT FOOD AND EATING

1. It's okay if you don't want to or can't eat something.

2. Judging, scolding, or mocking someone for their food choices is not helpful.

3. Food is not a punishment or a reward.

4. Helpful or constructive feedback on food qualities or traits is encouraged and will not be punished.

5. Everyone accepts that adequate nutrition is critical and is the one area that is nonnegotiable. Efforts will be made to ensure that everyone eats a healthful amount of calories, vitamins, and minerals for sustaining life and growth.

THE FIVE TASTES

You may be familiar with the diagram of the human tongue that shows the different regions of taste buds, neatly grouped into four areas: bitter on the back, sweet front and center, with salty along the sides toward the front and sour along the sides toward the back. But it's not nearly as simple as that.

First off, a whole other taste receptor has been discovered since the research behind that diagram was concluded: umami. Secondly, scientists have found taste buds on the roof of the mouth, in the throat, even in the intestine. That said, four of those five tastes are a bit like a game of Rock Paper Scissors in that they counterbalance or counteract one another—and knowing how can be invaluable in the kitchen.

CHAPTER 2

THE FIVE TASTES

SWEET

A spoonful of sugar helps the medicine go down!
—MARY POPPINS *(1964),* FILM

We all know that sweet foods are ubiquitous, from desserts to empty-calorie-laden treats such as candy and carbonated beverages. While sweet may be one of the easier tastes to cater to, doing so without relying on mass-produced, processed foods that may not meet our nutritional needs is a challenge. Baking is something that I take great pleasure in, but not everyone enjoys it or has the time to bake with regularity. Also, without the preservatives, artificial ingredients, and sugar, the shelf life of homemade goods is often limited.

There are several recipes in this book for baked foods that are sweet, high in protein and fiber, balanced between complex and simple carbohydrates, and full of vital nutrients and minerals. (Check out Signature Cinnamon Scrolls, page 165.) The tangzhong method both increases the moisture content of breads without making them heavy and increases shelf life by up to four days.

TANGZHONG METHOD

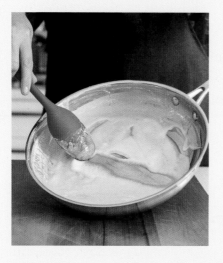

This Japanese technique uses the production of a cooked roux that is incorporated into bread dough. Adding additional liquid to the recipe and locking it in a small amount of existing flour in a gelatinized form made by the roux creates pockets of steam that release as the bread bakes. You can modify a yeasted bread recipe with this method, especially if you want a lighter, airy product. (This wouldn't be recommended for foods such as bagels, where you want a chewier or denser bread.)

To make this roux, reserve three to four tablespoons of the flour used in the recipe from the amount of flour called for.

Combine with two-thirds to three-quarters of a cup of water or milk and whisk until smooth in a small saucepan.

Heat over low heat, stirring often, until the roux resembles a loose, white paste. This stage is reached at 149°F, and the spoon will leave little trails on the bottom as you stir.

Allow the roux to cool to at least 98°F before mixing with the dough, to prevent the heat from killing the yeast.

The dough will be stickier and more elastic than you might be accustomed to if you are using it in a recipe you've made before.

On the flip side, if sweetness is something you are seeking to avoid, try one of the following:

- Add a squeeze of lemon or lime juice right before serving over the top of the dish after plating. Be careful not to accidentally dislodge some lemon or lime seeds onto the dish! Those are super bitter.

- Add one teaspoon of white wine vinegar or balsamic vinegar after you've incorporated your final seasoning component and while you still have five to ten minutes on the heat to help the flavors meld.

- Add water to the dish to thin it out, shortly after you've incorporated the final seasoning component. Start by adding one or two tablespoons of water and taste the effect this has on the flavor. Add one or two more tablespoons to dial in your desired taste.

- Substitute honey or maple syrup for white sugar. Both honey and maple syrup are a one-to-one conversion ratio (i.e., one cup of sugar can be replaced with one cup of honey or maple syrup). Decrease the liquid in the recipe by three to four tablespoons per cup of honey or maple syrup.

- Avoid caramelization of vegetables and aromatics by using a lower heat level in a smaller pan, in a process called sweating. This will allow you to soften the vegetables and bring out their flavors without browning them; browning them can accentuate the sweet taste.

BITTER

One who has never tasted bitter, does not know what is sweet.

—*GERMAN PROVERB*

Aversion to bitter flavors is one of the most common food aversions, especially in younger people. Yet, it remains difficult to describe or properly ascribe to foods.

Often, a person will be unable to convey what it is about some foods they dislike so much, and when it isn't attributed to texture or another more easily identified trait, it may be due to bitterness. The food averse may say that it's "sour," leaving others confused because they don't immediately connect bitterness to classic sour foods such as lemons. I've heard of smaller children with food aversions saying that bitter tastes "bad sweet," or using other constructed words and phrases to try to convey what's wrong with the food on their plate.

Many cruciferous vegetables (e.g., broccoli, Brussels sprouts, kale, cabbage, and collard greens) fall on the bitter spectrum but may not easily be identified as such. I know from personal experience that as a child I couldn't eat most of them, only being able to tolerate broccoli and cauliflower. But I was unable to articulate why and resorted to, "I don't like how it feels in my mouth," even though it wasn't really about the texture. My palate has grown in some ways, and now I enjoy cooked kale and asparagus. (The smell of Brussels sprouts still turns my stomach.)

An example of a food that is bitter in a sneaky way is tomato sauce, and especially homemade sauces that haven't been processed with additives. The truth is that a spoonful of sugar helps the *bitter* stuff go down.

Here are some ways to remedy bitter foods:

- Add a quarter to a half teaspoon of sugar or honey.
- Caramelize vegetables by sautéing them over slightly higher heat in a larger pan, giving ample space so that the vegetables don't steam and sweat. This will allow the natural carbohydrates and sugars in the vegetable to be pulled out and browned, highlighting the sweet flavors and offsetting the bitter.
- Add a sixteenth to a quarter teaspoon of salt—a natural balance to bitter.
- Add one teaspoon of fat (such as butter, olive oil, or coconut oil), which can reduce the amount of salt needed to offset the bitterness.

SALTY

Can that which is unsavoury be eaten without salt? or is there
any taste in the white of an egg?

—*JOB 6:6*

Salt naturally occurs in nearly everything we eat. As a preservative, it was instrumental in humankind's survival before we developed refrigeration. Without enough salt in our diet, we can become ill and even die. That said, too much salt can lead to ill health as well, which is more of a danger for those of us raised on the Standard American Diet, as we get most of our dietary salt through processed foods or food prepared in restaurants. Salt enhances the natural flavor of everything we cook, so adding it at every stage of the cooking process is a tried-and-true chef-approved method.

I'm going to let you in on a secret: One of the reasons many food-averse people fixate on a favorite boxed mac and cheese or will only eat pizza from a single source is that it's way saltier than most home cooks would ever prepare. It's a common joke in the hospitality industry that when a customer asks, "How is it so much better when you make it than when I make it at home?" the answer is that the cooks in the restaurant kitchen *don't love you* and are willing to add in as much fat and salt as it takes to taste amazing. The good news is that my recipes are geared toward making food taste good *without* overloading it with salt and butter.

But what if a dish is *too* salty?

Here's how to balance out salt:

- If you only need to temper the saltiness a little, add a pinch of sugar during the early stages of cooking and allow the flavors time to meld.

- Add half a teaspoon of something acidic, such as lemon juice or distilled white vinegar, along with half a teaspoon of sugar. You can add the lemon juice as a garnish at the final plating, but the vinegar and sugar should be added when there are five to ten minutes of cook time left, in order to allow the flavors to meld.

- If it's a soup, stew, or sauce, add a little liquid, such as water or broth, to thin it out. Check that the broth is sodium-free or you'll just be throwing accelerant on a fire, so to speak.

- Try a splash of heavy cream, but note that other creamy ingredients such as dairy-based butter or coconut butter can have the unintended effect of enhancing the flavor of salt. Rice milk, which has a naturally sweeter taste, is particularly useful (just be sure to avoid vanilla or other flavors); add one teaspoon at a time and then taste.

- Add a grain or carbohydrate to a soup or stew to absorb the salt. Rice, barley, or potato can both make food heartier and save an overly salty dish. Try mixing in a small amount, such as a half cup of uncooked rice, pearled barley, or diced potato, with one cup of water or sodium-free broth.

- Caramelization (see page 3).

SOUR

Sour is one of the flavors, along with bitter, that serves as a taste-based biological warning system. The human tongue is especially attuned to detecting sourness, largely because acidity and sour profiles are a by-product of food spoilage. Fruits and vegetables with a natural sour taste have adapted to protect their seeds from certain mammals, whose digestive tracts would destroy the seeds, but remain viable prospects for birds, who do not detect the sour taste and whose digestive tracts allow the seeds to remain intact for propagation.

Whether it's the mouth-puckering tartness of lemons or limes, the tang of sourdough or vinegar, or even the taste of melons or apples that just aren't quite ready to eat yet, sour food aversion makes a lot of sense.

There are several ways to neutralize sourness:

- If there is only a mild note of sourness, a pinch of sugar might suffice.

- Caramelization (see page 3).

- Add an eighth to a quarter teaspoon of baking soda to raise the pH level and eliminate acidity. Use sparingly, as too much can create an almost soapy bitterness in food.

- Add fats and salt (see page 16).

- Thin the dish with liquid, as you would with something that's overly salty (see page 18).

UMAMI

The debate rages on about whether umami, Japanese for a "pleasant, savory taste," should be included as the fifth taste. It might be the ephemeral nature of the flavor that leads to so many disagreements. It is difficult to describe exactly *what* umami tastes like. It's found in many cooked meats, fish, shellfish, broths, stocks, mushrooms, and fermented products, and its absence is often described as a "thinness" or lack of flavor. Salt is a critical complement to umami; without enough salt present, it remains nearly undetectable. Respectively, umami enhances the perceived presence of salt, so food manufacturers making low-sodium products will add ingredients like soy sauce or miso to create a tastier product.

To improve umami in a dish, try the following:

- Use broth or stock of any variety instead of plain water.

- Add one teaspoon of soy, fish, or Worcestershire sauce.

- In a soup or stew, add a couple of strips of crispy bacon or a bouillon cube. For a vegan option, tomato paste has a similar effect. Essentially, you are imparting flavors via a culinary cheat code. Crispy bacon gains strong umami flavor when the fats are browned, which happens rapidly due to the thin nature of bacon. The flavor remains even if the texture is altered by cooking in a moist medium. Bouillon is already long simmered or cooked, as is tomato paste, which is a tomato sauce cooked long enough to reduce the moisture content and concentrate the flavor.

- Use a longer cook time. Depending on the dish, if it's a soup or stew, sometimes ten to fifteen extra minutes is all the time you need to allow those flavors to deepen and become more complex. If it's a hunk of protein, you might add a quick sear to it for one minute under the broiler before slicing or serving. Just be watchful, because it can go from adding some color to being burnt rather quickly.

- Add a pinch of MSG.

MSG

Monosodium glutamate. When you read those words, do you feel a twinge of fear? There is a small amount of the populace that experiences adverse reactions to MSG (about 1 percent), but it in no way explains the vitriol and hostility aimed at this additive.

Like a lot of problematic things in the United States, this one is rooted in racism and xenophobia. By the 1950s, MSG was in just about every mass-produced food in the United States, referenced in the 1953 edition of *The Joy of Cooking* as "the mysterious 'white powder' of the Orient… 'm.s.g.,' as it is nicknamed by its devotees." With the ascension of China and Japan in the manufacturing and tech world from the 1960s to 1980s, so too did the alarmist concern over the usage of MSG arise. (Despite all that, it is still an ingredient in many packaged foods because it makes them, uh, delicious.)

CAPSAICIN/SPICY/PUNGENT

I'm going to add more heat to the five versus four tastes flame-war and say that both sides are wrong. There are six. Just as fruits and vegetables use bitterness and sourness as chemical warfare against predation that fails to propagate the species, they also use capsaicin. Think: hot peppers.

Capsaicin is a unique and necessary addition to a food-aversion tool kit because it's often a clear dividing line. My son loves spicy food, so much so that he could have a fixation on spice alone. He puts Tabasco or hot sauce on just about everything, whereas countless others with food aversion cannot abide it. They are capable of detecting even the faintest traces of heat or spice, and for them even black pepper (which doesn't have capsaicin but a similar compound) is unpalatable.

WELL . . . MAYBE SEVEN? EIGHT?

I am probably wrong, too. Recent studies in rats show that fats alter the bloodstream the same way the other tastes do, so it's quite likely there are in fact seven tastes and fat is one of them.

There is also the question of specific genetic reactions in folks who, for example, perceive cilantro and coriander as being "soapy" or "rotten" in taste and smell. The genetic component is present in as many as one in four people. Is cilantro a base taste?

Other scientists say that humans possess fourteen tastes, and still others say that the number is infinite.

CHAPTER 3

COLOR

Color preference or aversion in food is far from uncommon, with many autistic individuals preferring beige/yellow-colored foods. I can personally attest to this, as most of the food I prepare for myself falls within that color scheme. This is connected to the need for non-stimulating and consistent visual input, which is why I recommend that eating environments for autistic individuals or people with a stimulation/sensory disorder are in a neutral palette with as few distractions as possible. Limited sound or ambient white noise, low lighting, and air purifiers with odor-neutralizing functionality are other ways to make eating less of a challenge.

Let's go through the primary colors and their associated hues and ways to either eliminate or curate each one by modifying predominant ingredients. I encourage using a color wheel and the tips within each section to match everyone's food preferences as closely as possible. It is my goal to provide natural food coloring alternatives first; however, there are some instances where it's not possible to reach a desired depth of hue and maintain the integrity of the dish without a little help through chemistry.

When I need to, I prefer to rely on gel food colorings. They seem to give the best results in consistency and require using less than other options. I'd rather use less if it's not a natural ingredient, for no reason other than it's less likely to unbalance the flavor or texture components of the dish.

RED

As a midwestern child, I wasn't all that into red food. My experiences were limited to apples, watermelon, and tomatoes, and I was not fond of tomatoes with any kind of texture. I was aware of the existence of red bell peppers, largely from seeing them on commercials for local restaurant chain Romeo's Mexican Food and Pizza's fajitas ("Nacho typical restaurant!"), but I had never tried them.

If you are cooking for a red lover, there are a number of options for enhancing the spectrum of color that don't require artificial food coloring. Powdered beet root can provide a great warmth without changing the flavor much. If you use the beet juice, you can get an incredibly vibrant color, but it comes along with a very bitter pill. Well, flavor.

That being said, vinegar is sometimes necessary to set red coloring or make it pop. This is evident in red velvet cake, which frequently calls for distilled white vinegar to set the color and also to help activate the baking powder as a leavener.

Sometimes particularly sensitive palates will note a sour aroma or flavor in foods that have been altered toward red, even in dishes without vinegar added. This is largely anecdotal from my experiences cooking for food-averse children (and myself), but it can be helpful to add a pinch of baking soda to balance out the acidity if such complaints are voiced.

ORANGE

Thanksgiving, Halloween, and autumn are often associated with orange, and thankfully there are several foods that fall (ha?) into this hue without food coloring or dyes. You can also use orange hues to produce a more vibrant red with blending. Adding a quarter cup of cooled cooked sieved pumpkin with an egg yolk and omitting the white of a single egg along with the traditional four hundred grams of

00 flour and three eggs can render a great orange pasta without changing the taste or the texture considerably.

YELLOW/BROWN

As I mentioned, I love yellow food. My happiest memories around my childhood table involved a plate of yellow/brown: corn, mashed potatoes, breaded and fried meat, and a dinner roll. I'd go weeks with nary another color in sight. Beige is truly my comfort color when it comes to eating.

The yellow/brown color family is the easiest to prepare for, as it largely consists of starchy foods, which are a fairly safe bet for most of the food averse. If you need more yellow, turmeric is always an option. Especially in things like soups or breads, a half teaspoon of turmeric doesn't change the composition of the dish or add offensive flavors. In savory dishes like macaroni and cheese, dried ground mustard will darken the hue, enhance the flavors of the dish, and, when handled deftly (not more than three-quarters of a teaspoon), it won't be identifiable.

GREEN

To help the readers understand just how powerful a food aversion might be, my editor asked where the Green section of this book was when reviewing my manuscript. I then realized that I had completely omitted green, perhaps my least favorite food color, without even noticing the error until it was pointed out by someone else. Well, okay, then.

Working toward a green color palette is very achievable, as evidenced by Saint Patrick's Day celebrations; nearly any food can be green if you want it badly enough. Unfortunately, some of those brighter, vibrant hues are only attainable by using artificial food coloring. That being said, blended baby spinach leaves can produce a rich green in sauces, even in sweet foods, without fundamentally altering the flavor. Baby spinach doesn't bring much to the table flavorwise, so you can render down one cup of baby spinach leaves into two to three ounces of baby spinach paste and add a tablespoon at a time to the process to try to filter in the right color. As the spinach paste is mostly liquid, you will likely need to adjust the already existing liquids in the dish. Adding a teaspoon of lemon juice to the spinach paste can help brighten the color.

BLUE

To be honest, it's hard to make food intensely blue without using food coloring—at least, not without fundamentally altering the taste and texture of the food. Blueberries skew toward brown when cooked and incorporated into things like dough or sauces. The trick that can sometimes work is a little red cabbage juice (one to two ounces) and a pinch of baking soda—it can produce a brilliant blue color, but I've had somewhat hit-or-miss results with it. Err on the side of using less red cabbage juice, and any amount used will replace another liquid in the dish to keep the consistency the same as the recipe. Butterfly pea flower powder leans more toward the violet side but is a passable blue, and one to two teaspoons in a baked good or other flour-based dish can create some really neat color effects. That being said, check out Berry Swirl Cookies (page 174) for some fun treats.

INDIGO/VIOLET

The world really is your oyster if you love indigo and violet foods. Truly, the deck is stacked with two powerhouses of natural food coloring mentioned in the Blue section. Blue butterfly pea blossoms, in both flower and powder form, are an awesome ingredient that can create a violet that is nearly magical without contributing much by way of flavor. And ube powder, which is a dried and pulverized Filipino sweet potato, is a delicious addition to sweets with an underlying vanilla and subtle pistachio flavor while bringing a coloration that has to be seen to be believed. Ube powder is often available locally in Asian food markets, and if not an option in powdered form, it's possible that the Filipino sweet potato will be there in all its potatoey glory.

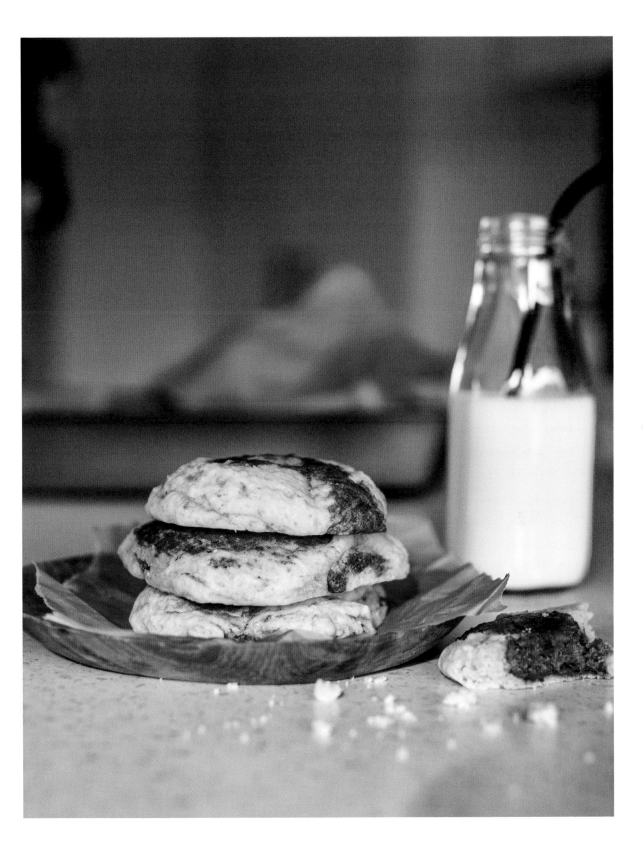

WHITE

There is a simple elegance to white food. Sometimes I like to stick to a monochrome white palette when I don't feel too hot physically. An upset stomach that might rebel against a plateful of different colors isn't as triggered visually by plain white rice. White can be a calm, safe harbor, and along with yellow/beige, this is an easy palate to cater to. So many of these foods fall within the starch category and readily adapt to food-averse tastes. A dense béchamel (see Glossary) can sometimes help put a patch on color woes if white is an acceptable hue, but only if sauces are acceptable to the tastes of the hungry.

BLACK

For the inner goth or emo kid, I'm going to include a single tip for naturally black food coloration. It's a classic that has been used in pasta for years: squid ink. It is often available in Asian and Italian/European–centric food stores, and sometimes even in your average supermarket. If there is a food that your loved one simply won't eat because of its coloration, if they are fine with black, you could try squid ink as the nuclear option. Plus, let me say, if you have a kid or loved one with food aversions and they are cool with trying the food black, they are awesome. They are my hero, and please reach out to me with stories and pictures because they should be celebrated.

CHAPTER 4

TEXTURE

For the food averse, there is nothing more dish-defining than texture. How something feels in your mouth can take a taste that you love or are neutral toward and make it fully unpalatable. Thankfully, changing the texture of prepared foods is the one area cooks have the most control over.

In each of the sections below, you'll find general guidance on how to avoid or enhance a certain texture, as well as some known offenders—foods with particularly bad reputations. This is another Rock Paper Scissors scenario; by adding the "opposite" texture, you can mitigate many undesired qualities. For example:

Texture Aversion—Add or Dial In

Crunchy—Soft, Smooth

Squishy—Smooth, Soft

Thick—Smooth

Chewy/Stringy—Squishy, Soft

CRUNCHY

This texture is defined by a firmness combined with a sound made when eating, and it's particularly polarizing among the food averse. Crunchy is the most tactile of food textures; each chew can be slightly different than the last, and you feel the vibration through your jaw, with variance in feeling to the roof and sides of your mouth and tongue. It can turn the experience of eating into sensory overload—or provide a focus of sorts. Crunchy foods that are sharp enough to cut your mouth, such as some breakfast cereals or snacks like tortilla chips, can cause trauma and reinforce the aversion. Others, such as crispy fried chicken, may not have the same expected pain response and may be a samefood even for those with an aversion to other crunchy foods.

If you want your food crunchy:

- Cut fibrous vegetables into slightly larger pieces, to retain natural crispness.

- If you are cooking a starch, cut as thinly as possible (e.g., such as a potato sliced wafer-thin before frying into chips).

- Always try to keep food approximately the same size and thickness, so that it all cooks at about the same rate.

- Whenever you bread and fry, make sure the process is dry-wet-dry: First coat the food in dry goods, like flour, then in an egg wash, and then back in a dry product (e.g., dried bread crumbs).

- When frying, use a frying thermometer to ensure that you are at the optimal temperature when you add food to the oil. The temperature will vary depending on what you're cooking and what style you're looking to achieve. For instance, tempura fried foods are often cooked in the 350°F range, while a French fry cooks at 325°F. Pay close attention to the recipe to ensure that you are at the optimal temp. All fried goods in this cookbook have the oil temperature listed.

- Don't overcrowd the pan, or the oil temperature will drop too fast and the food will become soggy.

- Add a pinch of baking powder into your dry goods when breading. It will significantly help in the crisping process.

- Use a cooling rack to allow fried foods to drain and to prevent them from becoming soft on one side.

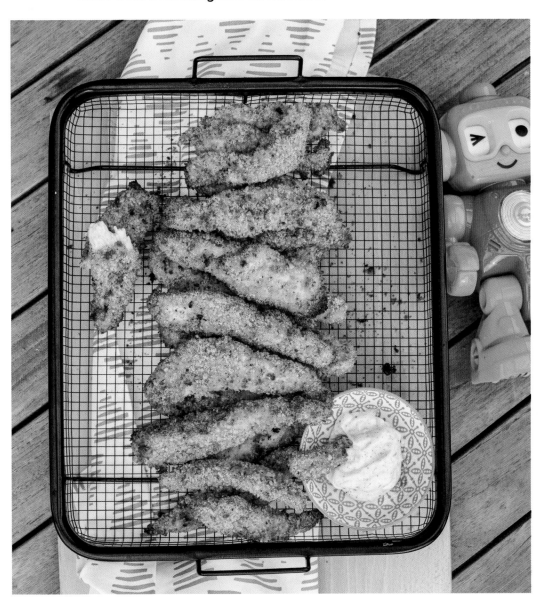

SQUISHY

CAVEAT: This particular trait is my culinary kryptonite.

Squishy foods are something of an amalgam of several other textures: soft with firmness that gives to pressure, and often slippery. Think of vegetables and aromatics such as uncooked diced tomato, large-diced onion, leek that has been quickly sautéed, and mushrooms cooked in sauce. Aromatics are the flavor base of French and Italian cuisine, in the respective forms of the mirepoix and soffritto (a medley of onion, carrot, and celery slow-cooked in butter or other fat). Because so much of Western and European chef culture is based on those two traditions, having a food aversion to squishy can be especially limiting in enjoying what is routinely called "fine dining."

If you want squishy food:

- Dice tomatoes or keep smaller vegetables whole to retain the juices.

- If the product has an innate crunch you are seeking to mitigate, cook it longer in a wet medium (broth, steam, or the like).

- If it's already squishy, either add it at the end of the cooking process or keep it raw (if food safe).

- Stewing, steaming, and sweating are your friends (see Glossary).

SOFT

These foods are yielding; they may have some firm qualities but they readily give way to the pressure of chewing. The inside of a baked potato, white sandwich bread, and pasta cooked past al dente are all examples of soft foods, which tend to be a safe zone among the food averse. While there are outliers (there are always outliers!), this texture is predictable and rarely associated with trauma from the experience of eating itself—that is, there is little chance of sensory overload or hurting your mouth when eating a piece of white bread. It's about the most benign way to gain sustenance.

When in doubt and I'm cooking something new for myself or another food-averse person, I aim to make foods softer and more homogeneous in texture.

Play it softly:

- If you are following a recipe that gives a range of cook times, err on the longer side.

- Oven fry rather than panfry or deep-fry.

- Dice or chop foods small.

- Enriched doughs and breads—meaning recipes that include butter, oil, milk, or eggs—are going to be a better bet.

THICK

This texture has a density in the mouth, such as a lentil soup or a hearty stew. It can be homogeneous or not in terms of one bite being the same as the last.

If you like thick foods:

- For a stew or a soup, add a thickening agent such as cornstarch slurry or a traditional cooked flour and butter roux, as follows:
  - One tablespoon cornstarch and two tablespoons cold water shaken aggressively in a mason jar provide enough thickening power for one cup of liquid—a slurry.
  - One tablespoon flour and one tablespoon butter cooked over low heat until it releases a fragrant, nutty aroma and slightly changes color will thicken one cup of liquid—a roux.

- Use an immersion blender to thicken a soup or stew without adding ingredients.

- Toss in a handful of uncooked quinoa, rice, or pearled barley with fifteen minutes or more remaining in the cooking process (the longer the better, as the grains will soften and meld into the background).

CHEWY/STRINGY

This category is defined by foods that have a density and firmness that require robust bite and jaw action to swallow. Many among the food averse have a pronounced gag reflex, which makes eating chewy and stringy foods a chore. Combined with any precedent of having choked on a chewy food, there is often an element of trauma to this particular aversion. As such, the reaction to this texture can be especially animated or heated.

Some examples are fibrous meat in solid cuts or on the bone that require cutting on the plate, sourdough or other dense breads, and tough vegetables such as snap peas or raw celery.

If you like chewy or stringy foods:

- The grain of any fibrous vegetable or meat is your friend, so cut with the grain to maintain long, unbroken fibers.

- Cook meat and vegetables low and slow, with indirect heat.

SMOOTH

This texture is homogenous in that there aren't any chunks or pieces that stand out or differentiate themselves. A preference for smooth is particularly common in the food averse. It's comforting to know what you're going to encounter with every bite.

The simplest comparisons would be creamy versus chunky peanut butter or tomato bisque versus chicken noodle soup.

Smooth tips:

- Dice tight and small.

- Cook over an even, medium heat with minimal turning or disruptions in the pan.

- Make sure you don't overcrowd your pan so that things cook at the same rate.

- Use a ricer for starches to achieve a consistent texture.

- An immersion blender will make short work of bigger pieces.

CHAPTER 5

AROMA

"Does it pass the sniff test?" isn't just a way of asking if a theory is credible. It's also how most of us first experience food before any other senses enter the equation, including sight. There is a reason that Realtors have been known to throw a batch of cookies in the oven before an open house. Our sense of smell is critical to our thinking process, memory retrieval, and a feeling of comfort. Smell is also a fundamental part of the experience of taste. This is one explanation for why there are so many examples of food aversions related to migraines, motion sickness, or pregnancy; each of those conditions is often associated with a heightened sense of smell. Autistics and people with attention-related neurodivergence often experience sensory overload with a less effective filter toward extraneous input and are bombarded with stimuli that can't be ignored. (Neurotypicals are much better at filtering out what isn't important, so the smell of what someone is eating three tables down, even if they don't like it, becomes less problematic as their brains focus on the plate in front of them.)

I can't tolerate buffets or family-style meals where I must serve myself. Sensory overload is a large part of this for me. When I'm standing in front of dozens of foods, even if I like three or four options, if the others make me physically ill to smell and

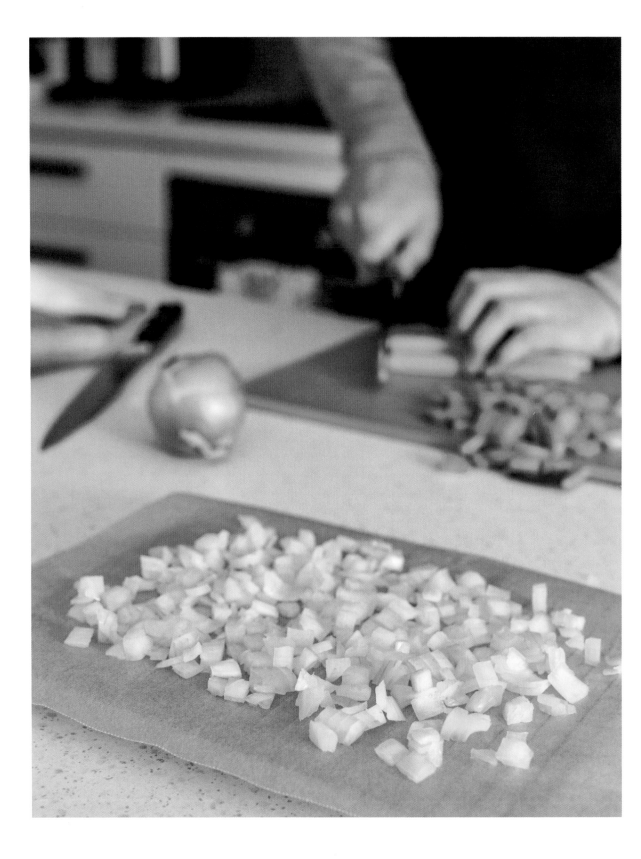

I'm inundated with traumatic memories… well, you can see why it becomes tricky. The outcome is that I grab a plate with one thing that I can tolerate and it's not enough to fill me up, so now I'm stressed out and close to a meltdown. I remember one time as a child, I grabbed a plate of sunflower seeds. Just scoops and scoops of unshelled sunflower seeds.

MINIMIZING FOOD SMELLS

The de facto remedy to cutting down food smells in the home is a good-quality air purifier. Even a tabletop HEPA-quality air purifier with replaceable filters and charcoal pre-filters can be had for approximately $50 plus the cost of upkeep (replacing the filters every one to three months based on usage). I find the low levels of white noise additionally helpful for blocking out outside sounds, and I keep a purifier in every room.

If an air purifier doesn't work for you, there are a handful of other options. While they are less immediately effective, they do help to prevent the accumulation of food aromas. Your scent-sensitive friends will thank you!

- A bowl of white vinegar next to the stove will neutralize alkaline odors; however, some people have an issue with the smell of vinegar itself. So play this one by ear (or nose).

- A small bowl of baking soda mixed with activated charcoal near the stove and a few strategically placed around the eating area is a surprisingly effective and scent-benign method. Replace the mixture every month to preserve efficacy. Placing these bowls near forced air vents and the intake is especially helpful.

- Improvise an inexpensive mechanical air filtration technique with a box fan, two pleated furnace filters, and some bungee cords. For around $20, it's a shockingly powerful solution. Be careful to place the filters on either side of the box fan properly, by being mindful of the arrows on the filters, which indicate the air flow.

Position the filters so that the arrows point in the direction that air flows through the fan, in one direction. If you can put the box fan in an open window so that it ventilates the kitchen air out of the home, you'll achieve the best results. If you can't put it in an open window, though, that's fine: Position the fan so that it is pulling the air away from the stove and ideally in the opposite direction of the dining area.

VINEGARY

A vinegar aroma can be mitigated by adding a pinch of baking soda when there are five to ten minutes left in the cooking process. This will allow the baking soda to neutralize more of the scent, and the soapy flavor that it can sometimes add will be minimized. If the vinegar aroma is more potent than desired in a sourdough (which will naturally have a tang to it), let the bread breathe a few minutes after slicing and before consuming. Sometimes adding condiments will bring out an intense vinegar aroma, and it can be helpful to give it a minute before bringing the sourdough to the table if the scent is problematic.

FISHY

Fish shouldn't smell excessively fishy; if it does, it could mean that it's close to its expiration date, and you might want to try something else for dinner (especially if the color of the fish seems off, it has a slimy film to it, or if it breaks apart too easily with handling while uncooked, all signs of food spoilage). If it just smells like fish, though, lemon or lime juice can cut through, as does rosemary. This can be done in a couple of ways. You can add a spray of fresh lemon or lime juice right before serving, and a whole sprig of rosemary can be left on the plate as a garnish. You could also squirt the dish before cooking with citrus and have the rosemary in the pan as it cooks, which is very helpful if you are panfrying in butter or olive oil.

ALCOHOL

Aside from dishes that actually contain alcohol, such as coq au vin or a flambéed dessert, you might be surprised to find that alcohol off-flavors are quite common in breads, especially in sourdough. In dishes that are alcohol predominant, such as the first examples, little can be done to help banish the boozy scent.

PUNGENT

Unfortunately there are some aromas that just cut like a knife. The spiky-skinned durian fruit, for example, has an aroma that has been compared to raw sewage or rotting flesh. The smell is so bad that in some places in Singapore and Malaysia it's illegal to eat it in public spaces. There is only so much that I can do or offer as a remedy for truly pungent scents. Open your windows and get the air moving in a cross breeze in and out of enclosed spaces. It's chemical warfare and all weapons are approved in clearing out the unwanted smells. Perfume-laden sprays, odor-neutralizing chemicals—do what you have to do. Just be safe out there.

CHAPTER 6

PLATING AND ENVIRONMENT

Location, location, location!

—REALTORS AND THE FOOD AVERSE

Where food is on the plate, how it's placed there in relation to other food, and where that plate is set have, fundamentally, the greatest impact on whether the food averse will eat that meal.

Imagine the best meal you've ever had the fortune to eat. Maybe it was surf and turf with new potatoes roasted in duck fat and garnished in slivered truffles, with a side salad of spring greens and a raspberry vinaigrette. And more truffles or something, I don't know—I'm not a foliage or fungi fun guy. Nothing could ruin your perfect meal if it's cooked expertly, right? What if it was served to you after everything was put through a blender? Or, you had to eat it in a truck stop bathroom? It may not seem as appetizing now.

If I'm served a delicious bacon double cheeseburger, but it is dressed in ketchup, mustard, lettuce, tomato, onion, and pickles, there is no removing the toppings for me. I can still smell them. I can still picture them on my food, even when

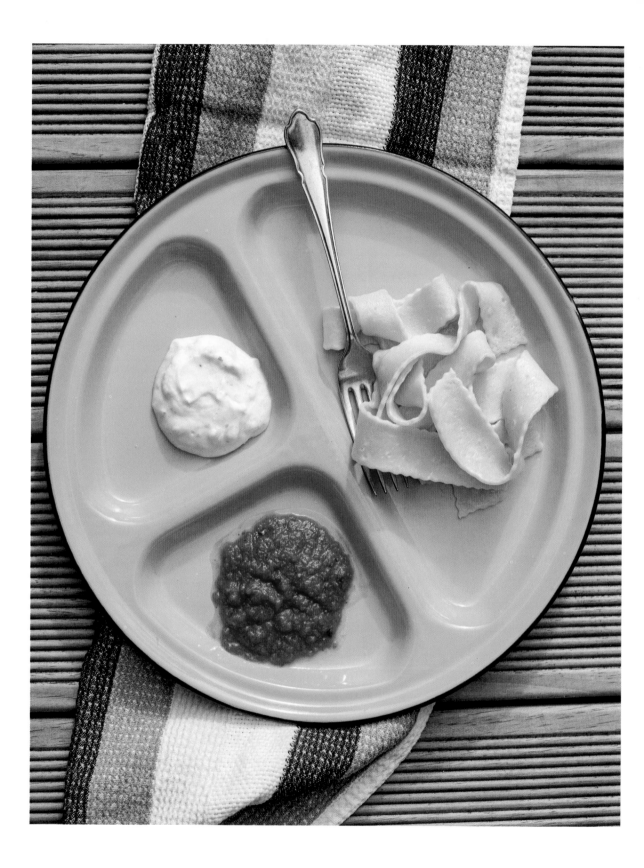

the offending ingredients are out of my line of sight. The traces of flavor have permeated the bun and the meat and cheese, like the haunting remnants of an invasive, colonizing, spectral salad.

TOUCHING PREFERENCE

"Mom! They're touching me!"

Undesired contact isn't just an issue for siblings; it's a common food aversion. I remember the Thanksgiving when I was in kindergarten and my grandmother made me a plate of food. I could barely look at it, much less eat it. The sweet corn had juice running into my mashed potatoes. The gravy from the mashed potatoes was on my turkey, corn, and roll. Cranberry sauce was on everything. I stood behind my chair and stared at the plate in horror. My mom took my plate and made me a new one.

Not wanting your food to touch is, frankly, logical. Juices can cause foods to become mushy, for example, changing the expected texture. Autistic people don't like unexpected phenomena; we find comfort in routine and pattern. There may even be a psychological and evolutionary advantage to not wanting your food to touch or revulsion to food not being what you expect. Before the invention of things like food safety protocols, either found in codified scientific principle or passed down by word of mouth as common sense or folk wisdom, determining what was safe to eat and how to safely prepare it was largely an issue of trial and error—and the error could lead to serious illness or even death. An enhanced physiological experience of repulsion when you take a bite of something that "shouldn't" be soggy might just have been the thing that saved you.

WHAT CAN I DO TO MAKE A MEAL MORE ENJOYABLE AND SAFER FOR MY ANTI-FOOD-TOUCHING FOLKS?

- Japanese bento, either as single-serve take-out or a home-packed meal, uses a partitioned and often stackable box that offers a practical and fun way to keep food separated.

- Cafeteria-style trays are an affordable and reusable method to prevent food from touching.

- Use smaller or individual plates or bowls for the sides and entrée.

- When bento boxes, cafeteria-style trays, or individual dishes aren't an option, careful serving and plating can mitigate some of the dangers of foods touching that shouldn't. Use a slotted spoon or colander to drain foods that have juices (e.g., kernel corn or green beans) before plating.

MIXED IN

For the longest time I was perfectly content with most of the ingredients of a fried rice if they existed in solitary confinement. I loved rice. I liked corn, carrots, peas, and green beans. I could tolerate water chestnuts on my plate, even if I wouldn't eat them. I was partial to scrambled eggs. If onions were present, I could banish them to a napkin with only a slight gag. I didn't hate soy sauce. But if one were to take all these things and combine them in the same pan, all bets were off. I couldn't eat it if my life depended on it.

This is one of the few areas where my food aversion has naturally evolved over time to allow items to be mixed and amalgamated, but I very much understand the need for things to remain in carefully curated culinary rows.

SAUCES/CONDIMENTS

To paraphrase Jerry Seinfeld, "I'm ketchup intolerant. I have no patience for ketchup, and I won't stand for it!" To be fair, I could say the same about mustard, mayonnaise, relish, pickles, horseradish, tartar sauce, and a number of other things that many consider to be kitchen staples. While I'd like to present this as a philosophical commentary on the purity of each dish, it's a simpler situation: I don't like how condiments taste. Like a cat who has been cruelly exposed to a cucumber, if condiments appear on my food uninvited, I too will recoil in fear.

TIPS:

- Serve sauces and condiments on the side.
- Properly seasoning food from start to finish will minimize the need for sauces and condiments.
- Many times sauces are used to offset overly dry food. The temperature guidelines for food safety have changed over the years, and investing in a good probe thermometer is a solid way to ensure that you are cooking your foods perfectly.

TEMPERATURE

I love hot tea and coffee. I enjoy iced tea and coffee. But if my hot beverage has cooled to room temperature, it's unpalatable. Very little demonstrates temperature of food preference better than that. When it comes to this category, there is a strong basis in culture and early exposure. I was raised in poverty. If something was cold, and it wasn't "supposed" to be, there was something wrong with it, implying that it wasn't cooked properly or thoroughly. Gazpacho, a cold, raw, blended vegetable soup from Spain and Portugal, is my idea of culinary torture. Soup isn't "supposed" to be cold.

Another example of mine is shrimp cocktail. I like breaded and fried shrimp,

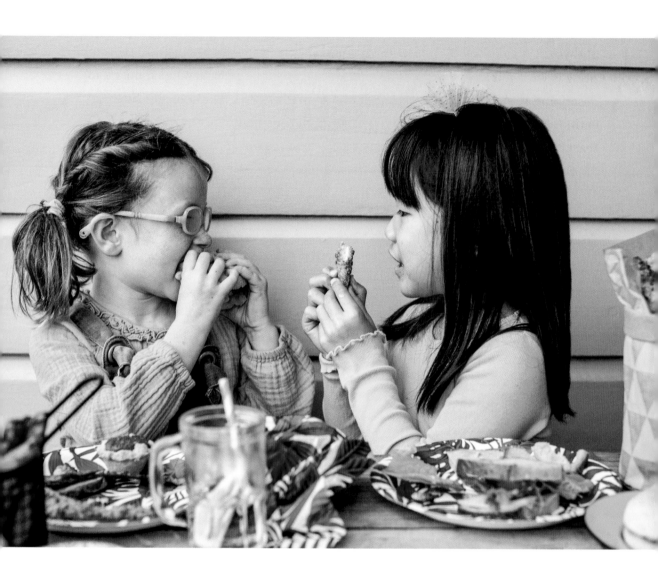

but I can't get over the revulsion I experience eating cold shrimp. My brain just knows that there is something *off*.

There are other factors involved in temperature preference. Autistics aren't always able to identify what their bodies are experiencing. We may know that something is wrong, but we aren't able to make the cognitive connection to labeling and describing it. As such, many of us have untreated cavities or tooth sensitivity, so eating something very cold or very hot can hurt, even if we can't communicate the reason why we can't eat it.

Suggestions:

- Most dishes should rest for at least five minutes after you take them off the heat. This goes for pizza, fried chicken, and mashed potatoes. Pretty much anything with a sauce that's an amalgam of other products (mashed potatoes) or that's a protein you've cooked with heat needs to set. Roasts or other large single pieces of meat you need to slice will have a carryover rise in temperature of five to fifteen degrees after you take them out of the oven and can take up to thirty minutes to reach internal equilibrium.

- If a soup is too hot, put an ice cube in it. This is especially useful if you need to temper flavors or thin it out as well.

TALKING DURING EATING

Norman Rockwell's famous *Freedom from Want* painting depicts a Thanksgiving celebration with a family seated around the table, with the viewer positioned at the foot of the table as congenial and merry faces look upon them. One can almost hear the murmur of conversation. It is largely seen as the traditional American family ideal. It may also depict a living hell for many autistics and other neurodivergent food-averse people.

I have auditory processing disorder and struggle to understand people if I can't read their lips, especially in scenarios with multiple people to track and extraneous background noise. Like many autistics, I experience discomfort with eye contact as well. Combined with a lifetime of predominately negative experiences at group meals, this scene is just begging for a meltdown.

Thankfully, of all the issues a food-averse person may encounter around the table, this is also one of the easiest to remedy. The scope of your approach is dictated by the needs of the person.

- Is their anxiety focused on their experience? In other words, if there were an understanding that they wouldn't be addressed during mealtime, or expected to participate in conversation, would this ameliorate or reduce their stress?

- If so, don't talk to them during mealtimes. Have an open and frank conversation with everyone around the table prior to serving, so that the food-averse person is not going to be addressed or spoken to and that there is no expectation of their participation.

- If ambient conversation is stressful, allow them to use noise-cancellation headphones or earplugs to reduce stimulation. If that doesn't provide enough relief, either commit as a group to enjoying a silent meal until they are finished eating or allow them to sit by themselves in a lower-stimulation environment.

It's understandable that you may feel some reservation on deviating from the image of what a family gathering "should" look like. I would encourage those who hew closely to those expectations to keep in mind that the most critical mission of this cookbook is to ensure that everyone has a trauma-free, nutritious, and health-ful relationship with food. While a quiet meal might break with the mold, keep this larger, loving picture in mind.

LOW-/HIGH-STIMULATION ENVIRONMENT

Sometimes, less is more. Think of some popular chain restaurants, especially those marketed as "fun": vibrant colors, brilliant lights, loud noises, piped-in music, multiple televisions tuned to different sporting events, and countless novelty signs, paintings, and decor... this is pretty much the perfect scenario for an autistic individual to experience a full meltdown. Put me in one, and I've got forty minutes, tops, before I can't stop tapping my feet and bouncing my legs, my hands shaking with anxiety. Likewise, place me in a room with no sound at all, beige walls, and nothing to occupy my senses, and sooner rather than later I'll start picking a fight with myself.

It's all about finding the comfortable balance for your loved one when it comes to their eating environment.

To find the middle road when it comes to low/high stimulation, start here:

- Eliminate extraneous sounds by turning off the television and radio.

- If there are busy or distracting decorations within eyeline, try to cover or move them.

- Place something on the table with a fascinating yet minimal tactile pattern, like carved wood or fabric.

- Use subdued, nonfluorescent lighting.

EATING SOUNDS

Imagine, for a moment, an orchestra. However, instead of the dulcet tones of the strings, the thrumming of the brass, and the haunting woodwinds, you're hearing the scraping of utensils on plates, rhythmic steady chewing of food, and periodic swallowing of drink. You hear this musical tableau every time you sit to eat with a group of people, and you are unable to tune it out.

Unfortunately, there is little others can do to create a more harmonious experience at the dinner table. Unless the group in question struggles with table manners, they are more than likely already chewing with their mouths closed and following the general niceties of polite society. The food-averse person who is triggered by eating sounds, however, has especially attuned senses. It's almost a superpower. (If there were a market for knowing when someone is quietly eating a snack in another room, it would pay dividends.)

My recommendations for minimizing the intrusiveness of eating sounds are similar to those for talking around the table:

- If possible, use noise-cancellation earbuds or headphones. If those are outside the budget, try regular headphones playing music that the food averse enjoys. Soft foam or swimmer's earplugs are an even less expensive sensory-reducing option.

- Any of the above makes it highly unlikely that the food averse will be able to participate in conversation, so a preliminary discussion about expectations would be helpful.

- Try setting a white-noise machine in the room where everyone is eating; talking might still be an issue, but this can mitigate other extraneous noises.

- If needed, arrange for the food averse to eat in solitude. While this is a last resort, it should remain on the proverbial table to ensure that they are getting adequate nutrition instead of avoiding mealtimes altogether.

CHAPTER 7

CULINARY TRICK SHOTS

Let's imagine some scenarios: You have a tried-and-true baking recipe and your loved one goes and develops celiac disease. The nerve of them. Now, you've got to try to make your cinnamon rolls gluten-free.

You're in the process of moving and your worth-its-weight-in-gold stand mixer is lost. After applying a generational curse to those responsible, you've got to try to make bread by hand. Like a barbarian.

Your kid has decided to go vegan to reduce their carbon footprint and out of genuine compassionate regard for living creatures. Honestly, you think you raise children right. Now you've got to make lasagna without egg, cheese, or meat.

This section will give you some guidance on adapting a recipe to gluten-free, baking without a stand mixer, and converting a meal to vegan or vegetarian.

Also included are some time-saving and safety tips.

GLUTEN-FREE BAKING—YOU CAN TAKE OUR GLUTEN, BUT YOU CANNA TAKE OUR . . . BREAD!

Gluten-free baking isn't a simple one-to-one conversion, unfortunately. You can't just replace wheat flour with rice flour and call it a day. There are frequently changes to liquid ratios, required additions such as xanthan gum to bind and emulsify, and bulking leaveners to increase crumb rise and softness. It's pretty much a unique beast when compared to "standard" baking and would require an entire cookbook to teach you how to masterfully adapt any recipe.

That being said, here are a few tips to keep in mind when making gluten-free bread.

> At each stage of the cooking process, right up to coming out of the oven done, it will be wetter and stickier than you will feel comfortable with if you are a "routine" baker.

> After the first rise, you want to handle the dough gently. Whereas I'd recommend you just straight up punch my sandwich dough like it owes you money after the first rise, you want to use a lubricated flexible spatula to kind of coax the dough to deflate a bit before ushering it to the loaf pan with the care one would normally reserve for a white-glove delivery service, rarefied instruments, or handling ancient manuscripts in the rare books section of the library.

> If shelf life were measured like a vehicle in miles per gallon, this bread would be clocking yards per gallon. You've got a day to consume your gluten-free delights before they turn into a pumpkin. Scratch that, you can possibly eat a pumpkin. Alternatively, you can slice and freeze the bread to extend the shelf life.

MAKING DOUGH BY HAND—TAKING A STAND WITHOUT A STAND MIXER

So you don't have a KitchenAid stand mixer. I know they are expensive, and if you are on the fence about whether they are worth it, please allow me to say: THEY ARE. (Sorry, don't mean to yell.) If you can afford the price of admission, a stand mixer is going to change your life in the kitchen. They are culinary beasts of burden that will be passed down from generation to generation.

That said, you can certainly bake without one. I've included some no-knead baking recipes that won't even be a chore (page 139). Otherwise, it's just mind over matter. Well, muscle over matter.

If you are weirded out by the feel of dough as you knead it, or simply want to improve your cleanup time, using food-safe latex or non-latex disposable gloves is my go-to tip. If you have food aversions and are trying cooking seriously for the first time, I recommend that you get gloves from the get-go. And give them a go.

If you aren't familiar with kneading dough by hand, use a large mixing bowl placed on a dry dish towel on a counter. This will provide extra traction for the bowl, so it doesn't slide all over the place.

Start by adding and mixing liquids and then add the dry ingredients slowly, with a big mixing spoon to get everything incorporated. Once you have everything mixed together, it's time to Hulk "smash."

Look at the shaggy mass of dough in the bowl like a round letter that you are folding, mentally dividing it into four quadrants. Grasp a quadrant and fold it back over to the other side of the dough and press down firmly with your palm, rotate the mixing bowl a quarter turn, grasp the next quadrant, and repeat the process. Continue this until the dough is smooth and elastic, kind of like Play-Doh. This can take up to ten to fifteen minutes, so watch some funny TikToks or something to pass the time.

To see if you've adequately developed your gluten (meaning, it's stretchy enough to get you the results you want), attempt the Windowpane Test. Grab a few ounces of dough. Flatten it out a bit into a rectangle, pinch a corner, and pull it gently away from the center mass of the rectangle to see if you can stretch it thin enough to see light through it without it tearing. If you can, it's ready for a rest and a rise. You're probably ready for a rest, too!

VEGAN/VEGETARIAN OPTIONS—MEATLESS ME IN THE MIDDLE

Whatever your reasons for not eating meat or animal by-products might be, your needs should be respected and honored. As such, all the recipes in this book are easily adjusted to be either vegan (no animal by-products at all) or vegetarian (no meat).

Some tips for adapting any baking recipe to make it vegan:

- One-to-one replacement of butter with coconut oil.
- A quarter-cup replacement of unsweetened applesauce for one egg.
- One-to-one replacement of dairy milk with your favored milk.
- To replace milk for thickening, one teaspoon of cornstarch or powdered arrowroot.
- Reduction of the baking temperature by twenty-five degrees Fahrenheit.

RIGHT IN THE THICK OF IT—THE IMMERSION BLENDER

Given the price point and countertop footprint of the stand mixer, it can be understandable that it's a luxury that not all can afford. If possible, however, invest in an immersion/stick blender. If you are food averse or you cook for those who are, it gives you true control over the finished texture of sauces and soups. No-frills models can be obtained for around $20, but the convenience and ease of mind a culinary-grade miniature boat motor offers is priceless.

SAFE VEGGIE TIME-SAVERS

Once you've created a list of safe vegetables, making your own prepackaged and frozen sachets is a quick and effective way of cutting down on cooking time. I recommend making an aromatic blend and a medley for soups, stews, or stir-fries. By bagging a few ahead for the week, you can make meal adjustments on the fly.

In my household, we are okay with the standard mirepoix of onions, celery, and carrots if they are diced very fine and break down well with cooking. Freezing diced vegetables will also assist in the aromatics becoming homogenous and innocuous in texture as they are cooked. My vegetable medley includes sweet corn kernels, whole green beans, and peas. You can up the carrot content or add broccoli florets or remove tricky items as needed.

My Safe Aromatic Blend is two white onions, two celery stalks, and one medium carrot diced fine.

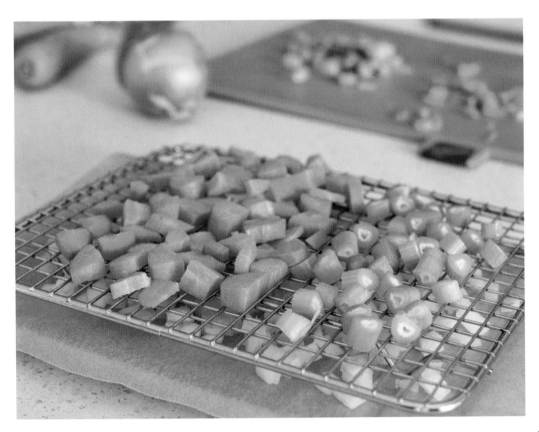

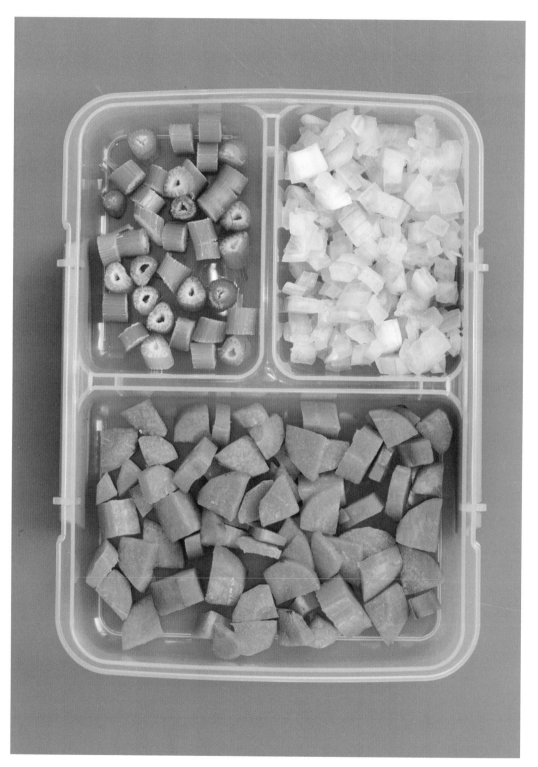

NO HEROES IN THE KITCHEN

It's happened to all of us: We're dicing veggies and we run into the knob end of an onion or whatnot that's got lots of salvageable product remaining on a very unwieldly platform. We have been cutting food all day and haven't cut ourselves once, not even close. Maybe you've been practicing your knife skills and are feeling confident that you can save that last measure of an inch of aromatic. I would, at this time, like everyone to ingrain the title of this section in their brains and say it out loud if you must as the situation arises: **There are no heroes in the kitchen.**

Whether you get that extra bit of food won't matter in the vast scheme of things. A month from now, the likelihood that you'll be reflecting on disposing of two tablespoons of unprocessed celery that you might have been able to save is slim. And even more important, as someone who has cut off the tip of their right index finger during a careless moment of kitchen bravado with the dreaded mandolin, even if I think, "Wow, I wish I had spent more time cutting that carrot last week, because that soup could have used more carrot," I can also guarantee you that I have more frequently waxed over the desire to have not cut off my fingertip that one time.

I simply cannot stress this enough: Any feat you think is super cool and worth the risk to your intact fingers, unburned epidermis, or unblanched face... *isn't*.

Step away from the cutting block and compost that quarter cup of vegetation. Use a ladle to spoon a manageable amount of scalding-hot milk into your roux as you whisk it. You aren't storming an entrenched castle, and you don't need to risk your precious skin to disfiguringly molten liquids. Take the time to work in the kitchen safely and leave the gambling to opening loot boxes in *Fortnite*.

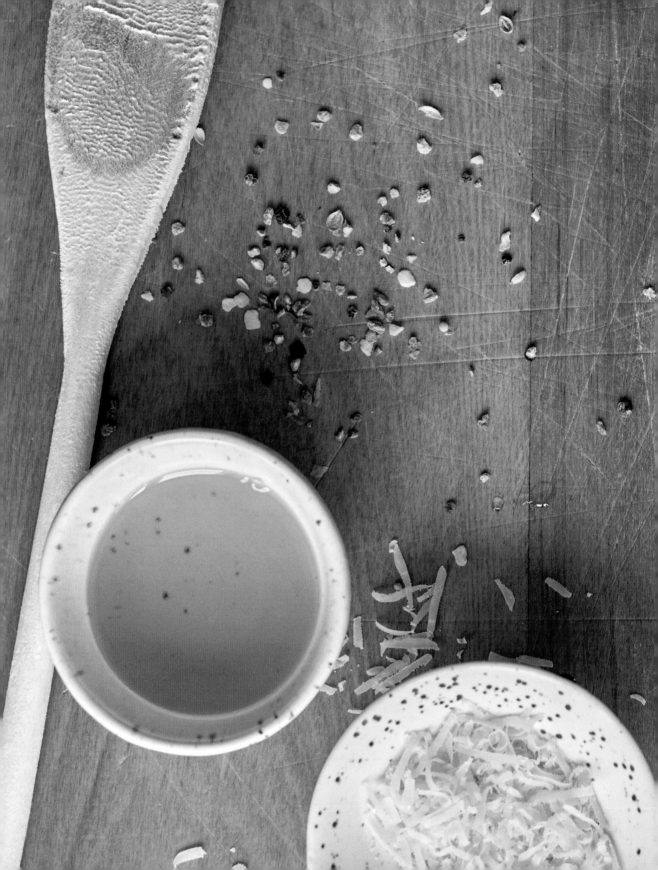

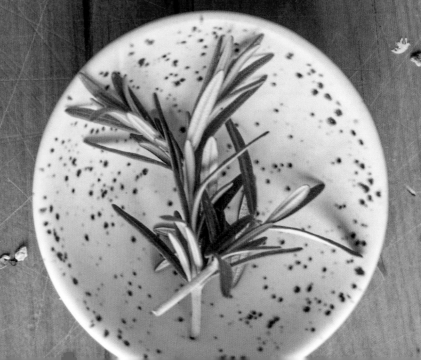

CHAPTER 8

RECIPES

BREAKFAST

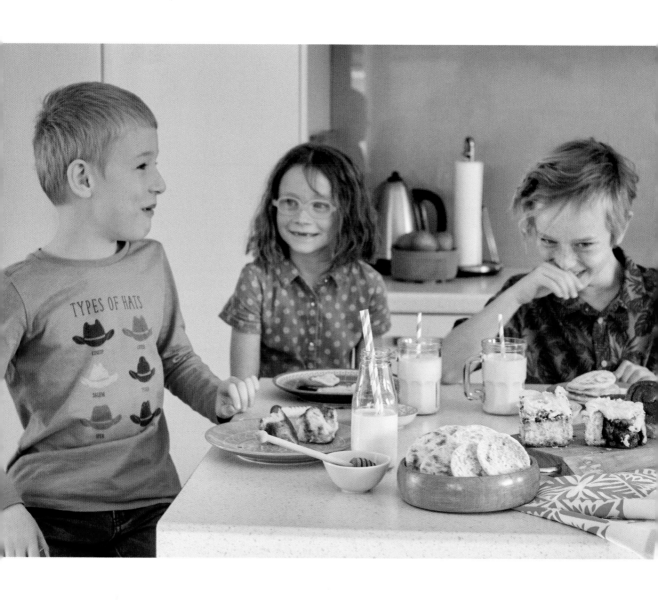

Crumpet/English Muffin/Biscuit Hybrid

I don't have a better name for these, but it's literally what they are. Maybe a Breakfast Bread Hybrid is a good name for it, but it's meant to be something that's super easy to make, that isn't so persnickety as biscuits, and that's a no-brainer to make egg sandwiches from. I prefer to use crumpet rounds to cut them, so I can use the same size form to poach eggs.

SKILL LEVEL: EASY

COLOR: WHITE, YELLOW/BROWN

KEYWORDS: BREAD, CRUNCHY, SOFT, VEGETARIAN

Makes about 18 breakfast breads

1 cup buttermilk, or ¾ cup plus 2 tablespoons whole milk plus 2 tablespoons distilled white vinegar

1¾ cups all-purpose flour, plus more for the pastry board

1 tablespoon light brown sugar

1½ teaspoons kosher salt

1½ teaspoons baking powder

1 teaspoon baking soda

2 tablespoons melted unsalted butter

¼ cup cornmeal (optional) (see Note)

EQUIPMENT

Measuring cups

Measuring spoons

Mixing bowls

Whisk

Spatula

Pastry board

Rolling pin

Tea towels

Large skillet or griddle

3½-inch cookie cutters or crumpet rounds

Serving bowl or basket

STEP 0 (OPTIONAL): If making your own buttermilk, take a measuring cup and add 2 tablespoons distilled white vinegar and pour enough whole milk into it to make 1 cup. Set aside for 5 minutes.

RECIPE CONTINUES

STEP 1: In a large mixing bowl, combine the flour, brown sugar, salt, baking powder, and baking soda and whisk together until well incorporated. Drizzle the melted butter over the top of this and mix it around a bit. Pour the buttermilk on top of the mixture and use a spatula to stir until a messy, clumpy, somewhat sticky ball forms.

STEP 2: Toss a bit of flour onto the pastry board and turn out the dough, putting a bit more flour on top. Use a rolling pin to smooth out the dough and help it come together into a pliable texture, using a bit more flour when necessary to keep it from sticking to the rolling pin or the pastry board. Try not to overwork the dough so it won't get too tough. Roll this dough into a rectangle about ½ inch thick at most. Cover with a tea towel and let rest for 5 minutes.

STEP 3: Heat a large skillet or griddle over medium-low heat. Use a cookie cutter or crumpet round to cut the dough into as many breakfast hybrids as you can get, rolling the remnants of dough back together to ½ inch in thickness up to two more times. Any more and the dough becomes too tough. When you've finished cutting out all the breads, it's time to start cooking.

STEP 4: Without overcrowding the pan, throw the little bread discs down and let them sit without touching them for 4 minutes on each side before turning over. Remove from the pan and cover with a tea towel in a bowl or basket. The leftovers can be stored in a zipper storage bag on the counter for up to 2 days, or frozen for up to 3 months.

NOTE

The discs will seem on the dry side before frying and that's okay—there is no need for oil in the pan, although you can coat them in a little cornmeal if you'd like before frying to keep them from sticking. However, this is associated with a slightly acrid aroma/flavor, as sometimes described by those who don't like English muffins. Split nicely with a fork and toast up with cool little nooks and crannies.

The Best Omelet

Omelets are perhaps the best way to illustrate what the carryover phenomenon is to children and people with less experience in the kitchen. If you are making an omelet and it's fully cooked in the pan, when you serve it, it's going to be rubbery and nearly inedible, because the eggs retain heat and continue to cook even after you take the pan off the heat and place on the plate. While some people like their omelets to be a little on the firmer side, we can account for this in preparation. If you are following this recipe for someone who prefers it firmer, add another 10 to 12 seconds to each stage on the heat. Otherwise, this prepares a "classic" omelet, with the middle of the dish the texture of a soft-set custard.

SKILL LEVEL: EASY

COLOR: YELLOW, WHITE

KEYWORDS: TOUCHING, SALTY, SOFT, GLUTEN-FREE, VEGETARIAN

Makes 1 large omelet

1 tablespoon salted butter

3 large eggs, at room temperature

Salt and freshly ground black pepper to taste

⅓ cup of your favorite shredded cheese

EQUIPMENT

Medium skillet or omelet pan

Mixing bowl

Fork

Spatula

STEP 1: Heat a medium skillet over medium-low heat for 3 to 4 minutes. Add ½ tablespoon of the butter.

RECIPE CONTINUES

STEP 2: Crack the eggs into a mixing bowl and add salt and pepper. Use a fork to agitate the eggs and mix the egg whites and yolks together, with tight figure eight patterns, being careful not to incorporate too much air by keeping the tines pointed down and attempting to mix without causing a lot of disturbance on the surface of the egg (this helps prevent a rubbery texture).

STEP 3: Add the eggs to the pan and gently jiggle the pan in a circular fashion, while using your spatula in a figure eight pattern going the opposite direction from the direction you're moving the pan. Do not actually scrape the bottom of the pan—you are simply guiding the eggs to curdle in the proper way. Do this for 50 seconds on the heat. Remove the pan from the heat.

STEP 4: Add the cheese to the center of the eggs and use the spatula to fold the eggs over the cheese (shaped like a capital D), while tilting the pan away from you to help it slide more easily. Add the remaining ½ tablespoon butter and place back on the heat for 35 seconds. Remove from the heat, sprinkle with more salt and pepper to taste, and serve promptly.

NOTE

If you are making an omelet on an induction range, the process changes. Because the heating element changes so rapidly when you take the pan off the surface and the heat is so gentle without ramp-up time, you want to heat the pan over medium-high heat and work a little faster while it's on the heat. It might only take 30 to 40 seconds of jiggling the pan with the figure eight pattern. Pull the pan off the heat long enough to fold the eggs over any ingredients you placed in the center, and place back on the heat for just another 30 seconds, until you can hear a little bit of a sizzle as the edges of the egg brown or you physically see a change in color. Pull the pan off the heat and wait for about 10 seconds before folding it over again onto a plate. Wait a minute before eating and the carryover temperature will finish it off perfectly.

The pace feels a little frantic with an induction surface, but I've come to prefer to make omelets on them. The heating scheme (higher and faster versus low heat and a bit more handholding) feels more forgiving with a larger window of success than traditional gas or electric.

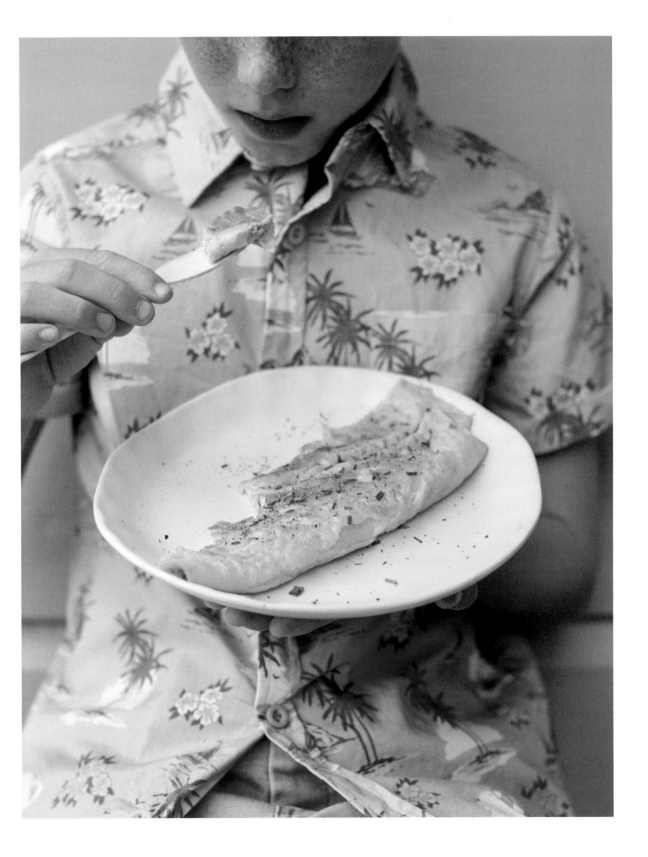

Egg Rounds

Perfect shape for egg biscuit sandwiches by using crumpet rounds. You can cook them soft or fry them hard, catered to the tastes of the hungry.

SKILL LEVEL: EASY

COLOR: WHITE, YELLOW/BROWN

KEYWORDS: SALTY, CRISPY, SOFT, GLUTEN-FREE

Makes 4 egg rounds

1½ teaspoons salted butter

4 large eggs

Salt and freshly ground black pepper to taste

Crumpet/English Muffin/Biscuit Hybrid (page 65), split

Sliced cheese or bacon, for topping (optional)

EQUIPMENT

Large griddle or skillet

Crumpet rounds

Cooking lid for medium pan

Spatula

Butter knife

STEP 1: Heat a griddle or skillet over medium-high heat. Place the crumpet rounds in the pan, and divide the butter evenly among the rounds. Crack an egg directly into a crumpet round. Crack some salt and pepper onto the egg. Repeat with the other three eggs. Go ahead and crack your knuckles if you're someone who does that, just to keep the momentum going.

If runny yolks are desired, leave the yolks intact. If no yolks are desired, break the individual yolks with the butter knife. Cover the crumpet rounds with the lid of a cooking pan. Cook for 1 to 2 minutes for slightly runny yolks. Cook for 3 minutes for hard fried eggs.

STEP 2: Remove the egg and round together with the spatula when the desired doneness is achieved. Place directly on split breakfast hybrid bread. Top with some cheese, bacon, or other desired accoutrements.

Gavin's Vanilla Shake

This is a modular recipe crafted for a Twitter mutual who asked for some alternatives for their child who loves vanilla. It's a portable meal that's soothing on the stomach and provides healthy protein and nutrition, and the incorporation of probiotics can help balance out a tummy prone to unease. It can be enjoyed immediately in the morning, or it will keep in a thermos until lunch with a cold pack. The consistency of this shake can be anything from a thick confection to nearly indistinguishable from a glass of milk with the adjustment of the use of ice cubes. More liquid additions mean a thinner final product.

You can add some chocolate syrup or malted milk powder for a different take. The use of ube powder (see Indigo/Violet on page 26) will provide a vibrant purple color with a bit of sweetness and nuttiness. Alternatively, favorite flavors found in frozen fruit might tilt the balance of scales toward your targeted palette/palate.

> SKILL LEVEL: EASY
>
> COLOR: WHITE, OPTIONAL (ANY)
>
> KEYWORDS: SMOOTH, COLD, SWEET
>
> ───────────
>
> Makes two 8-ounce shakes

1 tablespoon cold-soluble gelatin (see Note)

1 cup rice milk (or other shelf-stable milk alternative)

4 ounces probiotic vanilla or plain yogurt

¼ teaspoon vanilla extract

⅓ to ½ cup ice (depending on desired thickness) (optional)

EQUIPMENT

Measuring spoons

Measuring cups

Blender or food processor

Thermos (optional)

Cold pack (needed if packing in a thermos to go)

RECIPE CONTINUES

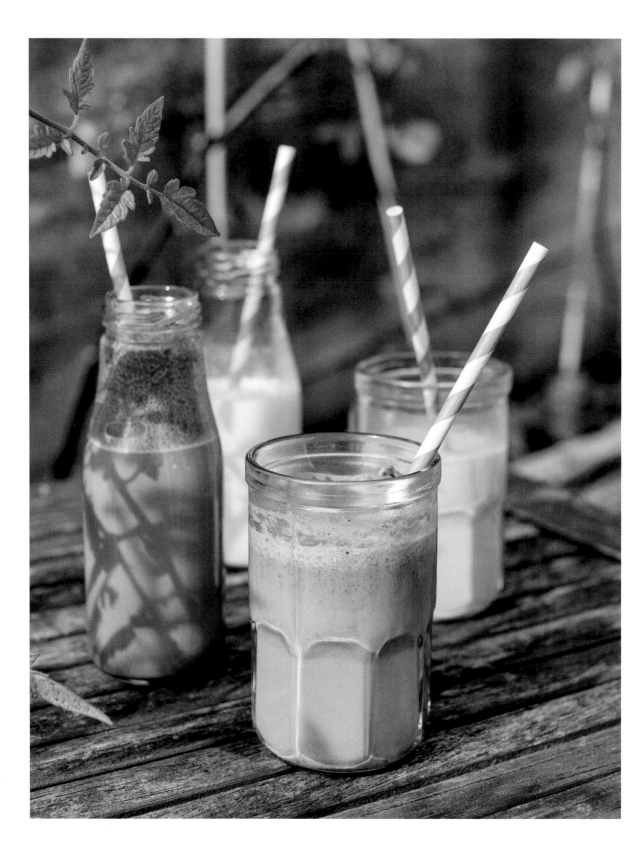

STEP 1: Put the gelatin, rice milk, yogurt, and vanilla in the bowl of a blender and pulse until smooth. Without the ice, it will be the consistency of melted ice cream. If a thinner, milklike consistency is desired, add the ice and pulse until smooth.

STEP 2: Either drink now or put in a thermos with a cold pack and it can be enjoyed at any time. Just be sure to shake your thermos heartily before drinking to ensure that it's well blended and hasn't settled throughout the day.

VARIANT: Purple Shake

As the base, but with 1 teaspoon ube powder added in Step 1.

VARIANT: Chocolate Shake

As the base, but with 2 tablespoons of one's favorite chocolate syrup added in Step 1.

VARIANT: Banana Shake

As the base, but with 1 peeled fresh or frozen banana added in Step 1. Will be thicker than standard.

VARIANT: Berry Shake

As the base, but with 4 ounces fresh or frozen favored berries in Step 1. Will be thicker than standard.

NOTE

This recipe calls for cold-soluble gelatin, which isn't the same as cold-blooming gelatin. It's a little harder to find, and you might need to resort to Amazon or some other source with far-reaching fingers. However, it makes all the difference. "Normal" gelatin softens first in cold but dissolves in hot fluid, resetting to firmness as the goods cool. For an ideal shake with the best consistency, the rarer cold-soluble version is required. Otherwise, it's grainy.

Buttermilk Pancakes

A quick meal that is taste packed and nutrient dense. Pancakes are the bane of many ill-prepared cooks, but with a little planning you can make sure that everyone eats delicious hot cakes of light, fluffy divinity at the same time.

SKILL LEVEL: EASY

COLOR: YELLOW/BROWN, WHITE

KEYWORDS: SOFT, HOT, SWEET, VEGETARIAN

Makes about nine 6-inch pancakes

3 cups buttermilk, or 2½ cups plus 2 tablespoons whole milk plus 6 tablespoons distilled white vinegar

2 cups all-purpose flour

2 teaspoons baking powder

1 teaspoon baking soda

1 teaspoon kosher salt

3 tablespoons honey or sulfur-free molasses

4 tablespoons melted unsalted butter, plus 1 tablespoon for the griddle

2 large eggs, at room temperature

1 teaspoon vanilla extract

Cooking spray (optional) (see Note)

EQUIPMENT

Measuring cups

Measuring spoons

Mixing bowls

Whisk

Microwave

Mixing spoons

Baking sheet

Aluminum foil

Large griddle or skillet

Ice cream scoop or ladle (optional, for dispensing) (see Note)

Spatula

Oven mitt

STEP 0 (OPTIONAL): If making your own buttermilk, add 6 tablespoons distilled white vinegar to a 3-cup measuring cup and top with whole milk. Set aside for at least 5 minutes.

STEP 1: Combine the flour, baking powder, baking soda, and salt in a large mixing bowl and whisk until combined. Place the honey in a small measuring cup and warm in the microwave for 10 seconds at 50% power. Add 4 tablespoons of the butter and stir until fully combined. If it's still too cold, place back in the microwave for 10 seconds at 50% power until it's a liquid.

STEP 2: Preheat the oven to 170°F and place a baking sheet lined in foil inside. Preheat the griddle to medium-high. It's ready when it's water-dancing hot (see Tip, page 76). Lightly beat the eggs with the buttermilk. Add the buttermilk to the flour mixture along with the butter and honey and whisk together until it's just combined. You don't want rivers and tunnels of loose flour, but lumps and clumps are perfect, and it will be rather thin. At the very last, stir the vanilla through with three quick rounds of a mixing spoon.

STEP 3: Put a little butter on the griddle. Using an ice cream scoop, pour the batter in a steady, single motion without moving the ice cream scoop around too much from about six inches off the surface of the griddle. A consistent motion will ensure a consistent pancake. Cook on one side for about 2½ minutes before turning over with a spatula. There should be lots of little bubbles around the outside of the pancake. Cook for 1½ minutes on the other side before removing from the griddle. Place on the warmed baking sheet in the oven—be sure to use an oven mitt so as not to burn your hand—and cover the pancakes with a single layer of loose foil.

STEP 4: Give the batter a quick stir with the whisk before repeating the process above until your good and honorable service is complete and you either get down to a few "silver dollar" sizers or do what I like to do and make one last massive beast of a pancake.

NOTES

I prefer to use an ice cream scoop to pour the batter. If you are using one to divvy up the pancakes, give the inner surface a good spritz with cooking spray. If not, a ladle is a good option, as is a ½-cup measuring cup. Either way, get those tools nice and lubricated with the cooking spray.

I like to stack similar quality and browned pancakes together on the baking sheet so it's easier to serve when the whole batch is cooked.

TIP: WATER-DANCING HOT

If the surface of your skillet or griddle is hot enough that when you cast a drop of water on the top, it immediately pops and jumps from the landing spot, your surface is to temperature!

LUNCHTIME

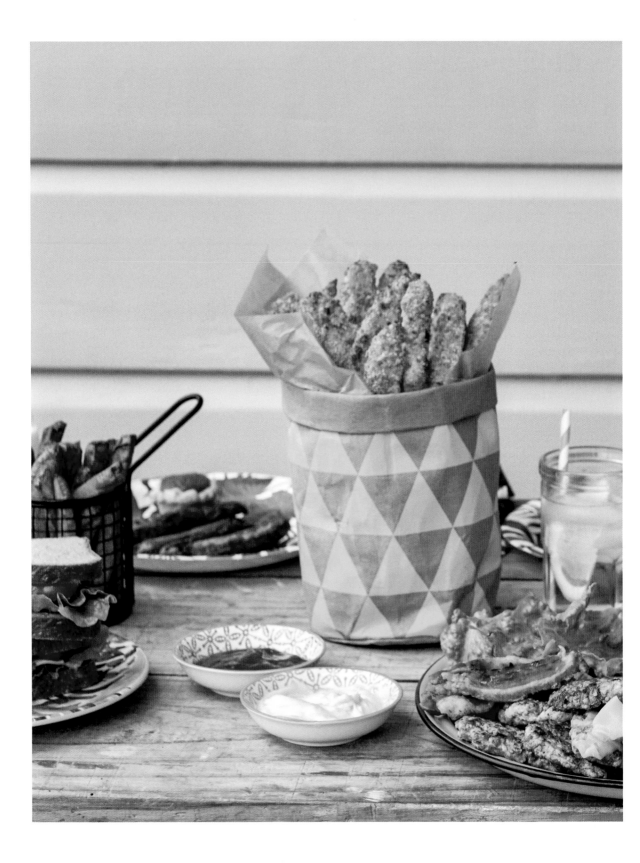

Chicken Fingers

Yes, we are all aware that chickens don't have fingers. It's a misnomer. A delicious misnomer.

SKILL LEVEL: INTERMEDIATE

COLOR FAMILY: YELLOW/BROWN

KEYWORDS: SALTY, CRUNCHY, JUICY (HOT, COLD, OR ROOM TEMPERATURE)

Makes 6 servings (about 12 "fingers" total)

1½ cups whole wheat flour

1 teaspoon baking powder

1½ teaspoons kosher salt, plus more to taste

1 teaspoon freshly ground black pepper

1½ pounds skinless, boneless chicken breasts sliced into "fingers" of about the same size, or precut tenders

2 large eggs

1 tablespoon non-skim milk

Vegetable oil, for frying

EQUIPMENT

Measuring cups

Measuring spoons

Freezer bags

Kitchen knife

Cutting board

Fork or whisk

Shallow bowl or pie pan

Cookie sheet

Aluminum foil

Latex-free disposable gloves (to prevent batter hand!)

Deep-frying skillet

Candy or frying thermometer

Long-handled kitchen tongs or large slotted spoon

Cooling rack over a cookie sheet

STEP 1: Mix the flour, baking powder, and half of the salt and pepper in a gallon-size sealable freezer bag.

STEP 2: Season the chicken with the remaining salt and pepper.

STEP 3: Lightly beat the eggs and milk in a shallow bowl or pie pan and place the egg mix in a second freezer bag.

RECIPE CONTINUES

STEP 4: Prepare a foil-lined cookie sheet to hold the battered chicken tenders, and put on your gloves.

STEP 5: Add one-third of the chicken to the freezer bag with the flour mixture and seal it. Lightly shake the bag and cover the chicken evenly.

STEP 6: Open up the bag and remove the chicken, shaking the excess flour off, and put the floured chicken in the egg bag and seal it. Lightly shake the bag to coat the chicken in the egg mixture.

STEP 7: Unseal it and remove the chicken and place it back in the flour bag. Repeat Step 5.

STEP 8: Place the now twice-floured chicken on the foil-lined cookie sheet and repeat Steps 5 to 8 for the remaining two-thirds of the chicken. Remove the gloves.

STEP 9: Place the chicken on the tray in the refrigerator to rest for at least 30 minutes.

STEP 10: Heat the oil to a depth of ¾ inch in a deep-frying skillet over medium heat until it reaches 365°F to 375°F on the candy thermometer.

STEP 11: Carefully place one-third of the chicken in the hot oil one piece at a time with tongs or a large slotted spoon and allow to cook on one side for 6 to 8 minutes, until golden brown. Don't overcrowd the chicken. Turn the chicken to the other side with the tongs or slotted spoon and allow to cook for another 6 to 8 minutes. The thicker the pieces of chicken, the longer it will take to cook all the way through.

STEP 12: Place the fried chicken on the cooling rack over a cookie sheet. Repeat Step 11 twice for the remaining chicken. Sprinkle the chicken tenders with more salt if desired.

Italian Sausage and Potato Soup

This hearty, flavorful soup was my son's favorite meal growing up. It's simple and warming and offers an opportunity to introduce texture in a nonthreatening manner. I recommend that the potatoes are diced a little larger and the kale is kept in bigger sections, so that either can be removed if they're problematic.

SKILL LEVEL: EASY

COLOR FAMILY:
WHITE, YELLOW/BROWN, GREEN

KEYWORDS: SALTY, CRUNCHY, CHUNKY, SOUP, GLUTEN-FREE

Makes about eight ⅔-cup servings

6 strips of bacon

1 tablespoon extra-virgin olive oil

2 garlic cloves, minced

1 large white onion, diced

3 celery ribs, diced

4 large carrots, sliced

1 pound bulk Italian sausage

4 large starchy potatoes, cubed, skin on or off

5 cups chicken stock or broth

2 bay leaves

2 cups chopped kale

Herbs, such as oregano, thyme, rosemary, and/or tarragon, to taste

1 cup heavy cream

Grated or shredded Parmesan cheese, for garnish

Kosher salt and freshly ground black pepper to taste

EQUIPMENT

Plate

Paper towels

Large stockpot

Kitchen tongs or spatula

Kitchen knife

Cutting board

Measuring spoons

Garlic press (optional)

Strainer or colander

Measuring cups

Mixing spoon

Ladle

STEP 1: Line a plate with paper towels and have nearby. Crisp the bacon in a large stockpot over medium heat.

RECIPE CONTINUES

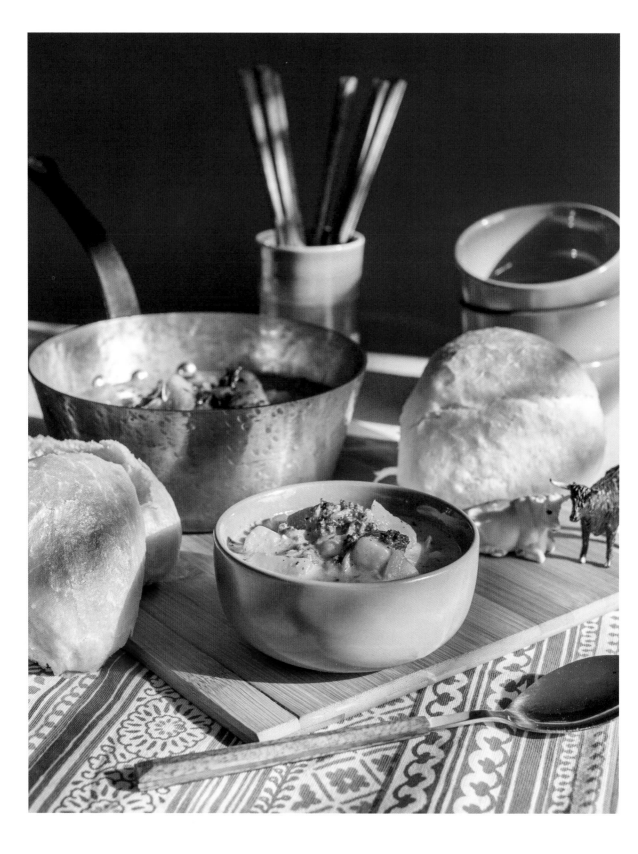

STEP 2: Remove the bacon from the stockpot and set it on the paper towel–lined plate. Drain all but 1 tablespoon of the bacon fat. Chop the bacon when cool enough to touch and reserve it for later.

STEP 3: Add the olive oil to the stockpot and reduce the heat to medium-low. Add the garlic and sauté for 30 seconds. Add the onion and sweat the onion and garlic for 3 to 5 minutes. Add the celery and allow to cook for 2 minutes. Add the carrots and allow to cook for 2 more minutes.

STEP 4: Add the Italian sausage and cook for about 5 minutes, until browned. Drain excess fat with a strainer or colander.

STEP 5: Combine the sausage and veggie mixture, potatoes, half of the chopped bacon (reserve the other half for garnish), chicken stock, and bay leaves to the stockpot and raise the heat to medium-high.

STEP 6: Bring the soup to a simmer and allow it to simmer for 25 minutes, uncovered.

STEP 7: Discard the bay leaves. Add the kale and allow to cook for 5 minutes.

STEP 8: Add the herbs.

STEP 9: Turn off the heat.

STEP 10: Stir in the heavy cream.

STEP 11: Ladle into bowls and top with the reserved chopped bacon and Parmesan cheese as garnish. Add salt and pepper to taste.

Multipurpose Soft Rolls

This is the bread and butter of the bread game. It is adaptable enough to be divided into seven portions for a delicious hamburger bun when given an egg wash and topped with sesame seeds. It can also be folded for hot dog buns or hoagies.

SKILL LEVEL: INTERMEDIATE

COLOR FAMILY: YELLOW/BROWN, WHITE

KEYWORDS: SOFT, SWEET, YEAST, VEGETARIAN

Makes 7 large rolls

1¼ cups body temperature (98.6°F) water, plus 1 tablespoon cool water

2 tablespoons honey

2¼ teaspoons active dry yeast

3 cups all-purpose flour, plus more for dusting a surface

⅓ cup whole milk

1 tablespoon unsalted butter, plus more for buttering a bowl, if using

Cooking spray

1 teaspoon kosher salt

2 large eggs—1 whole egg and 1 egg separated (use the egg white from the separated egg for the egg wash)

EQUIPMENT

Measuring cups

Measuring spoons

Stand mixer with the dough hook (optional; see Making Dough by Hand—Taking a Stand Without a Stand Mixer, page 55)

Small saucepan

Spatula

Large bowl

Kitchen towels

Cookie sheet or round pan

Parchment paper

Pastry brush

Cooling rack

STEP 1: Combine the warm water, honey, and yeast in the bowl of a stand mixer. Allow to bloom in a warm, draft-free place for 5 to 10 minutes, until frothy.

STEP 2: Make a tangzhong roux (see page 14) using ¼ cup of the flour and the milk. Add the butter, increasing the speed on the mixer to 3. Allow the

RECIPE CONTINUES

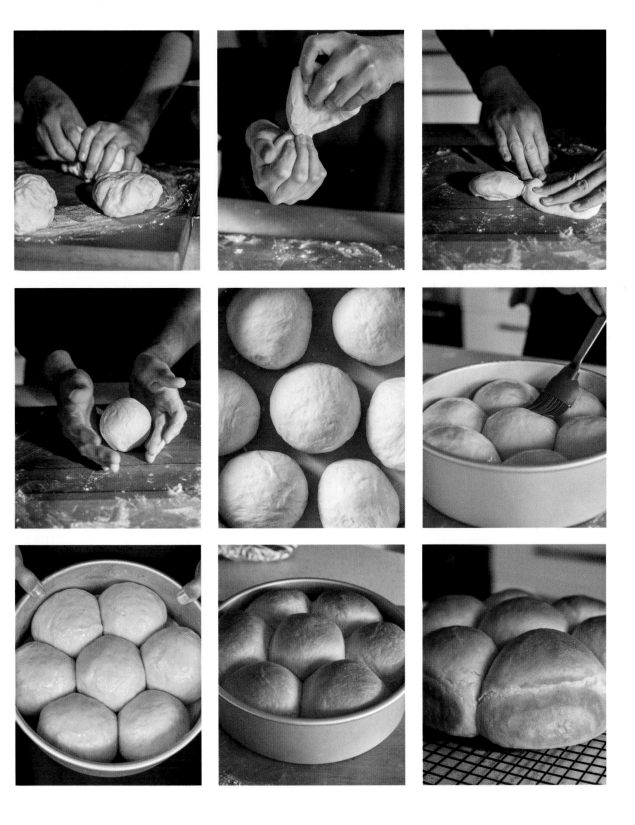

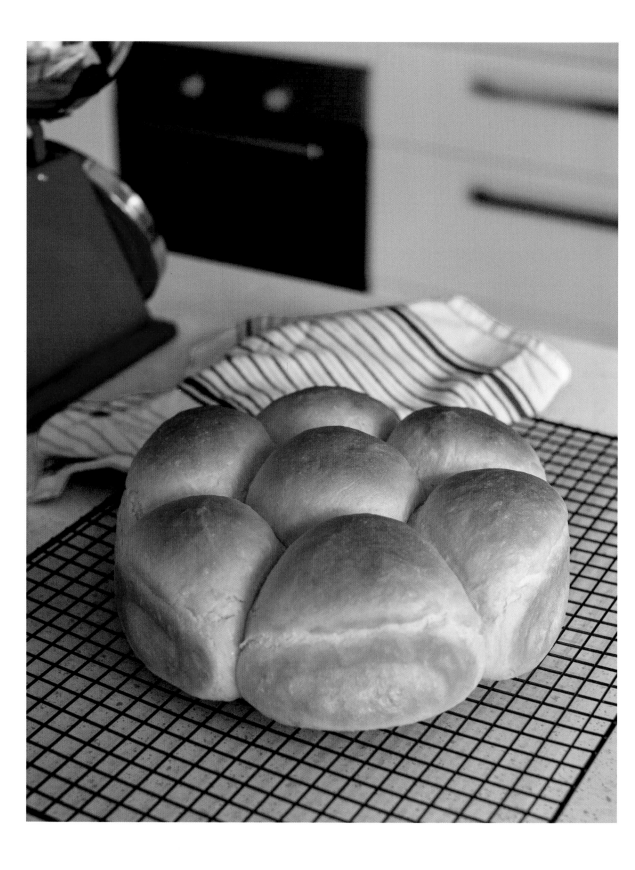

dough hook to work the dough for about 7 minutes, until it is smooth and elastic. It will still be sticky.

STEP 3: Spray a large bowl with cooking spray or butter the bowl lightly. Put the dough in the bowl and cover with a kitchen towel in a warm, draft-free place. Allow the dough to double in bulk, about 1½ hours.

STEP 4: Add the salt, whole egg, and egg yolk from the separated egg to the dough. Place the mixer on Stir or the lowest setting. Add the remaining flour, ½ cup at a time, slowly, allowing it to incorporate.

STEP 5: Cover a cookie sheet with parchment paper. Divide the dough into eight equal portions. Form the sections into balls on a lightly floured surface and rotate the dough balls clockwise while tucking with your pinky fingers to make a tight skin. Place them on the lined cookie sheet. Allow several inches of room between each bun. For dinner rolls, spray or butter a round pan. Place one dough ball in the center of the pan and arrange the remaining six balls evenly around the perimeter of the pan.

STEP 6: Cover lightly with a clean kitchen towel and allow to double in bulk, about 30 minutes, in a warm, draft-free place.

STEP 7: Preheat the oven to 375°F about 10 minutes into the second rise.

STEP 8: Brush the buns with the separated egg white mixed with 1 tablespoon of cool water. Place in the oven on the middle rack. Bake for 15 minutes and then rotate the cookie sheet or round pan for even browning. Bake for another 10 to 15 minutes, until golden brown.

STEP 9: Remove the cookie sheet or round pan from the oven and place the buns on a cooling rack until cool enough to handle.

Gluten-Free Soft Rolls

There are so many gluten-free flour blends out there, and I've made this recipe with some of the bigger brands with consistent success. Using honey helps provide a little more structure to the dough than you'd normally find in a gluten-free recipe. If you are a brand-new baker, gluten-free or otherwise, you will actually find it easier to make than if you have tons of "traditional" baking experience. Also, even if the flour blend you are using (or prefer) has xanthan gum, you really can't omit the amount in the recipe without a discernible loss in quality.

2¾ cups gluten-free flour blend (I prefer King Arthur's Gluten-Free All-Purpose Flour)

1½ teaspoons xanthan gum

2 teaspoons instant yeast

1 teaspoon kosher salt

1 cup warm water (must be under 110°F!)

¼ cup honey

2 tablespoons unsalted butter or coconut butter

1 large egg, at room temperature

Cooking spray

EQUIPMENT

Measuring cups

Measuring spoons

Cooking thermometer

Stand mixer with the paddle attachment

(optional; see Making Dough by Hand—Taking a Stand Without a Stand Mixer, page 55)

Mixing bowls

Whisk

9-inch-round cake pan or springform pan

Parchment paper

Ice cream scoop (for shaping the rolls)

Dish towel

STEP 1: Combine the flour, xanthan gum, yeast, and salt in the bowl of a stand mixer. Set the machine to Stir.

STEP 2: In a separate large bowl, combine the warm water, honey, and butter and whisk together. With the machine still on Stir, add the wet ingredients to the flour mixture in a slow and steady stream until all the dry ingredients are mixed with the wet ingredients. Add the egg and increase the speed of the mixer to 3 or 4, or Medium (whichever applies to your device). Knead for 3 minutes. It will be a big, wet, sticky, goopy ball.

STEP 3: Line a 9-inch-round cake pan or springform pan with parchment paper and spray with cooking spray. Scoop out seven rolls along the outer perimeter of the pan with an eighth in the center, with even space around them to allow for rising and baking—I like to use cooking spray on an ice cream scoop to help form the individual rolls. Cover with a clean kitchen towel and allow to rise in a warm, draft-free place for 1 hour.

STEP 4: Preheat the oven to 400°F. Bake the rolls in the center of the oven on the middle rack for 25 to 30 minutes, until the tops are golden brown. Remove from the oven, allow to cool for 5 minutes, then take them from the pan and pull the rolls apart. They may be served immediately.

Savory Piecrust

With a perfectly balanced piecrust, there are few mediums better suited to deliver a modular meal. This platform can deliver a banging vegan roasted root vegetable potpie, comforting classic chicken, or even a custom creation of your own that is crafted to meet your unique needs.

SKILL LEVEL: INTERMEDIATE

COLOR: YELLOW/BROWN

KEYWORDS: CRUNCHY, SALTY

Makes two single 9-inch-round piecrusts or tops and bottoms for three 4½-inch-round pans

½ cup unsalted butter, plus more for buttering the pans

½ cup lard

2½ cups all-purpose flour, plus more for rolling

1 teaspoon kosher salt

1 large egg

½ cup ice water

EQUIPMENT

Cookie sheet

Parchment paper

Cutting board

Kitchen knife

Plastic wrap

Measuring cups

Measuring spoons

Food processor or blender

Whisk or fork

Rolling pin

3 individual potpie pans or 1 (9-inch-round) pie pan

STEP 1: Line a cookie sheet with parchment paper. Cut the butter and lard into ½-inch cubes and place them on the lined sheet, making sure to leave space between the cubes to prevent sticking. Cover the pan with plastic wrap and place in the freezer for 30 to 45 minutes.

STEP 2: Place the flour and salt in the bowl of a food processor and press Pulse for 1 second.

STEP 3: Beat the egg and ice water together in a measuring cup.

STEP 4: Take the fats from the freezer and add them to the processor. Hit Pulse in 3-second bursts until the contents look like bread crumbs.

STEP 5: Slowly add the egg-water mixture to the dough while intermittently pulsing, until the dough combines into a tight ball. You may not need all the liquid.

STEP 6: Wrap the piecrust dough tightly with plastic wrap and put it in the refrigerator for at least 1 hour or up to 48 hours.

STEP 7: Place a sheet of parchment paper on a flat surface and lightly flour. Flour a rolling pin. Divide the crust into six equal balls. Roll out to ¼-inch-thick rounds.

STEP 8: Press gently into three lightly buttered potpie pans, reserving three rounds for the top crust. Or, use three balls to create a 9-inch crust. Place into a buttered 9-inch pie pan, reserving the remaining dough for the top.

STEP 9: If only using one 9-inch crust, press the extra crust into a buttered pie pan, cover in plastic wrap, and freeze for up to 3 months.

VARIANT: Sweet Piecrust

INGREDIENTS
Same as Savory Piecrust but:
Shortening instead of lard
1 tablespoon sugar

EQUIPMENT
Same as Savory Piecrust

Step 1: Line a cookie sheet with parchment paper. Cut the butter and shortening into ½-inch cubes and place them on the lined sheet, making sure to leave space between the cubes to prevent sticking. Cover the pan with plastic wrap and place in the freezer for 30 to 45 minutes.

RECIPE CONTINUES

Step 2: Place the flour, sugar, and salt in the bowl of a food processor and press Pulse for 1 second.

Step 3: Beat the egg and ice water together in a measuring cup.

Step 4: Take the fats from the freezer and add them to the processor. Hit Pulse in 3-second bursts until the contents look like bread crumbs.

Step 5: Slowly add the egg-water mixture to the dough while intermittently pulsing, until the dough combines into a tight ball. You may not need all the liquid.

Step 6: Wrap the piecrust dough tightly with plastic wrap and put it in the refrigerator for at least 1 hour or up to 48 hours.

Step 7: Place a sheet of parchment paper on a flat surface and lightly flour. Flour a rolling pin. Divide the crust into six equal balls. Roll out to ¼-inch-thick rounds.

Step 8: Press gently into three lightly buttered potpie pans, reserving three rounds for the top crust. Or, use three balls to create a 9-inch crust. Place into a buttered 9-inch pie pan, reserving the remaining dough for the top.

Step 9: If only using one 9-inch crust, press the extra crust into a buttered pie pan, cover in plastic wrap, and freeze for up to 3 months.

VARIANT: Gluten-Free Vegan Piecrust

INGREDIENTS

1 cup coconut butter

2½ cups almond flour, plus more for rolling

1 teaspoon kosher salt

¼ teaspoon baking powder

½ cup ice water

EQUIPMENT
Same as Savory Piecrust

Step 1: Line a cookie sheet with parchment paper. Cut the coconut butter into ½-inch cubes and place them on the lined sheet, making sure to leave space between the cubes to prevent sticking. Cover the pan with plastic wrap and place in the freezer for 30 minutes.

Step 2: Place the almond flour, salt, and baking powder in the bowl of a food processor and press Pulse for 1 second.

Step 3: Take the fat from the freezer and add it to the processor. Pulse in 3-second bursts until the contents look like bread crumbs.

Step 4: Slowly add the ice water to the dough while intermittently pulsing, until the dough combines into a tight ball. You might not need all the water.

Step 5: Wrap the piecrust dough tightly with plastic wrap and put it in the refrigerator for at least 1 hour or up to 48 hours.

Step 6: Place a sheet of parchment paper on a flat surface and lightly flour. Flour a rolling pin. Divide the crust into six equal balls. Roll out to ¼-inch-thick rounds.

Step 7: Press gently into three lightly buttered potpie pans, reserving three rounds for the top crust. Or, use three balls to create a 9-inch crust. Place into a buttered 9-inch pie pan, reserving the remaining dough for the top.

Step 8: If only using one 9-inch crust, press the extra crust into a buttered pie pan, cover in plastic wrap, and freeze for up to 3 months.

Chicken Potpie Filling

INGREDIENTS

¼ cup unsalted butter

2 cups Safe Veggies (as determined by Food Preferences Profile; see page 8), diced

1 teaspoon kosher salt

¼ cup all-purpose flour

2 cups chicken broth

½ cup whole milk

2 cups cubed roasted chicken

EQUIPMENT

Sauté pan

Spatula

Kitchen knife

Cutting board

Measuring cups

Measuring spoons

Step 1: Heat the sauté pan over medium heat. Melt the butter in the pan. Add the Safe Veggies and cook to specifications. Add ½ teaspoon of the salt.

Step 2: Add the flour to the pan with the veggies. Cook for 4 to 5 minutes.

Step 3: Add the chicken broth and milk to the pan and bring to a simmer. Cook for 7 to 9 minutes, until the broth mixture has thickened into a sauce and coats the back of a spoon.

Step 4: Add the cubed chicken to the sauce and incorporate the remaining ½ teaspoon salt.

VARIANT: Root Veggie Potpie Filling

SKILL LEVEL: EASY

COLOR: YELLOW, ORANGE, GREEN, PURPLE

KEYWORDS: SALTY, TOUCHING, MIXED IN, GLUTEN-FREE, VEGAN

Makes 8 large triangular wedge servings (if made in a 9-inch-round pan) or six 4½-inch potpie-pan servings

INGREDIENTS

2 tablespoons extra-virgin olive oil

1 tablespoon garlic, minced

1 large white onion, diced

1 teaspoon kosher salt, plus more for sprinkling

¼ teaspoon freshly ground black pepper,
 plus more for sprinkling

½ cup celery, diced

1 cup carrots, diced

1 cup potatoes, diced

1 large zucchini, diced

2 parsnips, peeled and diced

2 cups vegetable broth

1 bay leaf

2 tablespoons cornstarch

2 teaspoons herbes de Provence

Squash blossoms, for garnish (optional)

EQUIPMENT

Measuring spoons

Sauté pan

Spatula

Garlic press (optional)

Cutting board

Kitchen knife

Measuring cups

Small jar with a lid

Step 1: Heat the olive oil in the sauté pan over medium-high heat until the oil shimmers.

Step 2: Add the garlic and stir for 20 to 30 seconds. Add the onion and sprinkle with salt and pepper, stirring occasionally in the pan for about 7 minutes, until browned. Add the celery and carrots and stir to coat in oil, sprinkling with a bit more salt and pepper.

RECIPE CONTINUES

Step 3: Put the potatoes, zucchini, and parsnips in the pan along with the vegetable broth, bay leaf, 1 teaspoon of the salt, and ¼ teaspoon of the pepper and bring to a low boil. Reduce the heat to medium-low and allow to cook for 15 to 20 minutes, uncovered, until the vegetables soften.

Step 4: In a small jar with a lid, put the cornstarch and 2 tablespoons of cold tap water. Shake vigorously to combine. Bring the filling in the sauté pan back to a boil over medium-high heat and slowly stir in the cornstarch slurry. Discard the bay leaf and add the herbes de Provence. Turn off the heat.

All Together Now

INGREDIENTS	EQUIPMENT
1 recipe Savory Piecrust	Spoon
(either two 9-inch or six 4½-inch)	Paring knife
Chicken Potpie Filling or Root	Whisk or fork
Veggie Potpie Filling	Mixing bowl
1 large egg, for a wash	Pastry brush
	Baking sheet

Step 1: Preheat the oven to 425°F. Spoon the potpie filling on top of the bottom crust in the potpie pan(s) evenly.

Step 2: Top the filled potpie(s) with crust, pinching the dough sealed. Cut three ½-inch vents in the top.

Step 3: Whisk the egg and 1 tablespoon cool water in a bowl. Brush the tops of the potpie(s) with the egg wash.

Step 4: Put the potpie(s) on a baking sheet and bake for 30 to 35 minutes, until the top(s) are golden brown. Let stand for 5 to 10 minutes before serving.

Mashed Potatoes

A classic side dish that somehow can still go wrong in so many ways. A ricer is solid insurance against lumps, and adding just a pinch of salt at every stage of the cooking process ensures that you don't dance too close to the bland side. Roasting the potatoes as opposed to boiling them prevents your mashed potatoes from becoming a gloopy soup and helps them stand up on their own, both figuratively and literally. These mashed potatoes are lovely with a pat of butter or a dollop of sour cream, no gravy needed. (However, I did include my signature gravy recipe.)

SKILL LEVEL: EASY

COLOR: WHITE, BROWN/
YELLOW

KEYWORDS: SALTY,
SMOOTH, HOT,
GLUTEN-FREE

Makes five or six ½-cup servings

4 to 5 large starchy potatoes (like Russets)

4 tablespoons (½ stick) salted butter

2 to 3 garlic cloves, minced

½ teaspoon salt, plus more as needed

¾ cup sour cream

¼ to ½ cup heavy cream

Freshly ground black pepper

EQUIPMENT

Fork

Baking sheet

Oven mitts

Kitchen tongs

Cutting board

Sauté pan

Garlic press (optional)

Mixing spoon

Measuring spoons

Ricer

Stand mixer with the whisk attachment

Measuring cups

Chef's knife

STEP 1: Preheat the oven to 400°F. Wash and scrub the potatoes to remove any eyes or dirt. Prick the potatoes with a fork, penetrating about ½ inch in a

RECIPE CONTINUES

few places around the potato to allow steam to escape and for the potatoes to cook evenly. Place on a baking sheet and roast for 30 minutes. Remove the baking sheet from the oven using an oven mitt, and, with tongs, turn the potatoes to the other side, then place the potatoes back in the oven for another 30 minutes. Test with a fork to ensure that they are cooked thoroughly—if the fork goes into the potatoes with minimal resistance, they're done. Remove from the oven.

STEP 2: Melt the butter in a sauté pan over medium-low heat. Add the garlic and cook until fragrant, 30 to 45 seconds. Turn off the heat and add ½ teaspoon salt to the melted butter mixture. This will help the salt to distribute throughout the mashed potatoes evenly.

STEP 3: Use the ricer to extrude the cooked potatoes into the bowl of the stand mixer. Using the whisk attachment, turn on the mixer to Stir and slowly pour the butter mixture into the potatoes. Increase the speed to Low and add the sour cream a few tablespoons at a time. Once fully incorporated, add ¼ cup heavy cream. If the mixture looks too thick, add another ¼ cup. Increase the speed to Medium and beat until fluffy. Add pepper and more salt to taste.

VARIANT: Slightly Dirty Mashed Potatoes

This is a solid contender for someone who wants mashed potatoes with a little more substance to the bite. It still leans to smoothness but has less of the potential baby-food consistency that might come with perfectly homogeneous ricer-processed mashed potatoes. It's also easier to make if you don't have a ricer.

INGREDIENTS

Same as above, plus:

1 tablespoon extra-virgin olive oil

1 teaspoon kosher salt

½ teaspoon freshly ground black pepper

½ teaspoon garlic powder or onion powder

EQUIPMENT

Same as above, except:

Potato masher or two forks instead of ricer

Rub the pricked potatoes in the olive oil and toss in the salt, pepper, and garlic powder. Because the skins will be part of the finished dish, it only makes sense to season them now. Follow the above cooking instructions, and when cooked through, use a potato masher or two forks to smoosh completely, adding the cooked potatoes—skins and all—to the mixing bowl. Follow the rest of the directions above.

VARIANT: Filthy Loaded Mashed Potatoes

No longer a side dish, at this point, you're the star of the show, Spuddy. With vitamin-packed skins, bacon, and cheese, let's just face it: You're the head of household, Filthy Loaded Mashed Potatoes.

INGREDIENTS

Same as Slightly Dirty, except no olive oil or butter, plus:

6 strips of thick center-cut bacon

4 ounces (1 cup) shredded aged extra-sharp cheddar cheese

EQUIPMENT

Same as above, plus:

Skillet or griddle

Cooling rack

RECIPE CONTINUES

Step 1: Heat a skillet over medium-low heat. Place the strips of bacon in the hot pan and cook until they start to crisp on one side, 5 to 6 minutes. Turn over to the other side and cook for another 5 to 6 minutes. Put the cooked bacon on the cooling rack and reserve the bacon fat in the skillet.

Step 2: Toss the pricked potatoes in the bacon fat in the skillet before adding the salt, pepper, and garlic powder and roasting as above.

Step 3: Follow the directions above, crumbling half of the bacon and adding it after you've whipped the mashed potatoes, along with half of the cheddar cheese.

Step 4: Add the remaining bacon and cheese as garnish.

Gravy

This southern and midwestern American classic is essentially one of the Five Mother Sauces, specifically the velouté. Mastering this preparation will take one a long way in the journey to creating consistently good food.

SKILL LEVEL: EASY

COLOR: BROWN

KEYWORDS: SALTY, SMOOTH, HOT

Makes six ½-cup servings

2 cups broth or stock

½ cup pan drippings reserved from a roasted bird (see page 146) or 4 tablespoons (½ stick) unsalted butter

½ cup all-purpose flour

Salt and freshly ground black pepper

½ cup whole milk (optional)

EQUIPMENT

Measuring cups

Small saucepan or microwave-safe measuring cup

Medium saucepan

Whisk

Spatula

STEP 1: Heat the broth in a small saucepan over medium heat or in a microwave-safe measuring cup in the microwave until steaming, 1 to 2 minutes. Reserve until Step 3.

STEP 2: In a medium saucepan over medium-low heat, heat the pan drippings for 1 minute. Sprinkle the flour over the melted fat and whisk until smooth and clump-free. Cook the roux for 2 to 3 minutes, until it's lightly fragrant, stirring with the spatula and ensuring that you scrape the stuff off the bottom of the pan.

STEP 3: Adding about ⅓ cup liquid at a time, slowly pour the hot stock into the roux while whisking to avoid clumps. It should thicken very quickly. Once all the broth is incorporated, raise the heat to medium-high and cook

RECIPE CONTINUES

until the contents bubble, stirring constantly for about 5 minutes. Reduce the heat to low and cook for 5 to 6 more minutes to get rid of any raw flour taste. Add salt and pepper to taste.

STEP 4 (OPTIONAL): Heat the milk in a small saucepan or microwave-safe measuring cup for 1 minute. Gradually pour the milk into the gravy while whisking, for increased richness and a silky texture.

Perfect Smashed Cheeseburgers

I was cautioned against repeated use of the word *perfect,* but I had to keep this one. It truly is the perfect smashed cheeseburger for me. It contains the ideal amount of meat, cheese, and bun in one bite and knocks my socks off with flavor.

SKILL LEVEL: EASY

COLOR: YELLOW/BROWN

KEYWORDS: SALTY, RICH, HOT, TOUCHING

Makes 6 cheeseburgers

1½ pounds ground beef (no more than 85% lean, to not sacrifice flavor)

6 Multipurpose Soft Rolls (page 84), sliced in half

1 tablespoon salted butter, melted (optional)

Salt and freshly ground black pepper

1 tablespoon vegetable oil

12 slices cheese of choice

Preferred toppings, such as crispy bacon, sliced tomato, lettuce (optional)

EQUIPMENT

Griddle or large cast-iron skillet

Pastry brush (optional)

Food-safe latex-free gloves

Food scale

Measuring spoons

Burger press (or 2 heavy-duty metal spatulas)

Aluminum foil

STEP 1: Remove the ground beef from the refrigerator and keep covered for 15 to 20 minutes, to lose the chill.

STEP 2 (OPTIONAL): Preheat the griddle or skillet to medium heat, until a drop of water cast on the surface pops and sizzles (see Tip on page 76). Baste both halves of the split buns with the melted butter using a pastry brush. Carefully place the buns buttered side down on the griddle for about

RECIPE CONTINUES

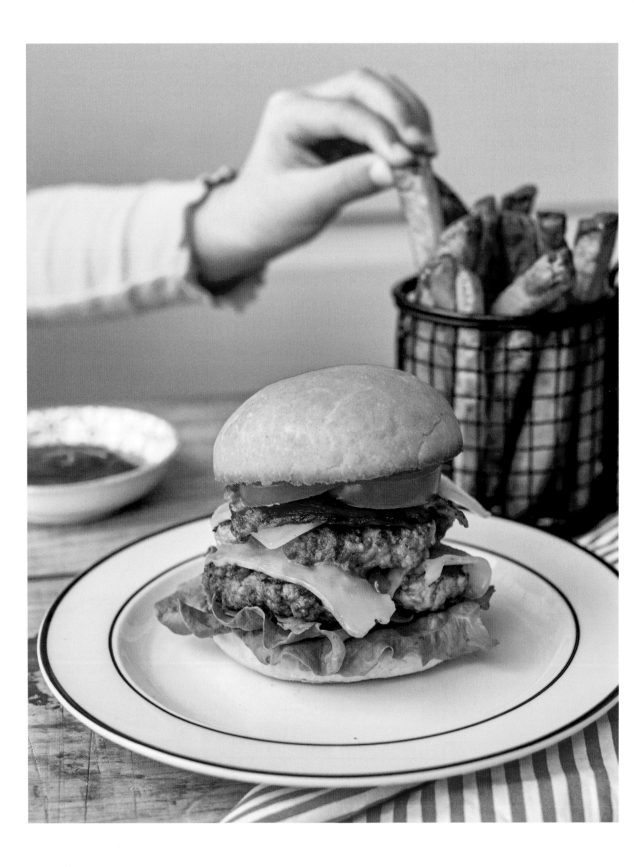

30 seconds, until they are golden brown. Fit as many buns as you can on the griddle without them touching one another. Set aside when finished.

STEP 3: Put on food-safe gloves and divide the ground beef into six loose 4-ounce portions. Sprinkle the portions with salt and pepper. Divide each of these portions in half and compress each portion lightly into a ball. There should be 12 balls.

STEP 4: Preheat the griddle or skillet to medium-high for 3 to 5 minutes, until a drop of water cast on the surface pops and sizzles (see Tip on page 76). Add the oil to the griddle and turn on the exhaust fan. Only work with 4 portions at a time, so as not to overcrowd the griddle. Place the balls on the griddle and press down with a burger press, or use two metal spatulas, with one applying pressure to the back of the other, until the beef is relatively thin (you want to get a good amount of surface contact with the pan while still holding the patty together for workability). For medium-well preparation, allow the burgers to cook for 50 to 60 seconds on one side before using the metal spatula to scrape them up and turn them over to the other side. There will be a good deal of smoke. Press the other side down the same way as before. Top each section with sliced cheese. After 50 to 60 seconds, scrape one of the sections and stack on top of one of the others. Stack the other portion. Remove the first two stacks from the griddle, being sure to scrape up the good bits. Set on a plate and tent with aluminum foil, to help preserve the heat. Repeat until all the burgers are complete. Place on the split buns, top with your preferred toppings, and serve.

Macaroni and Cheese

Pasta and cheese all piping hot and gooey, just carbs exploding in every mouthful. It's easy to understand why mac and cheese can be a samefood for so many!

SKILL LEVEL: EASY

COLOR: YELLOW/BROWN

KEYWORDS: SALTY, TOUCHING, HOT, MIXED IN, VEGETARIAN

Makes about twelve
½-cup servings

2 teaspoons salt, plus more to taste

1 pound uncooked macaroni

9 tablespoons unsalted butter

¾ cup all-purpose flour

4 cups whole milk

Pinch of grated nutmeg

4 ounces cream cheese

2 cups shredded cheese (about 8 ounces)

2 teaspoons soy sauce

1 teaspoon ground mustard

Freshly ground black pepper

1 cup fresh bread crumbs (optional)

⅓ cup shredded Parmesan cheese (optional)

1 teaspoon herbes de Provence (optional)

EQUIPMENT

Stockpot or pasta pot

Measuring spoons

Colander

Large saucepan

Spatula

Measuring cups

Microwave-safe measuring cup or small saucepan

Whisk

Kitchen knife

Cutting board

Casserole dish (optional)

Food processor or blender (optional)

Aluminum foil or casserole lid (optional)

STEP 1: Fill a stockpot or pasta pot with about 16 cups of water, place over high heat, and allow it to come to a boil. When boiling, add the salt to the water to flavor the pasta later. Cook the macaroni according to brand specifications and your family's taste. Drain thoroughly, reserving 2 tablespoons of the pasta cooking water to help thin out the cheese sauce.

RECIPE CONTINUES

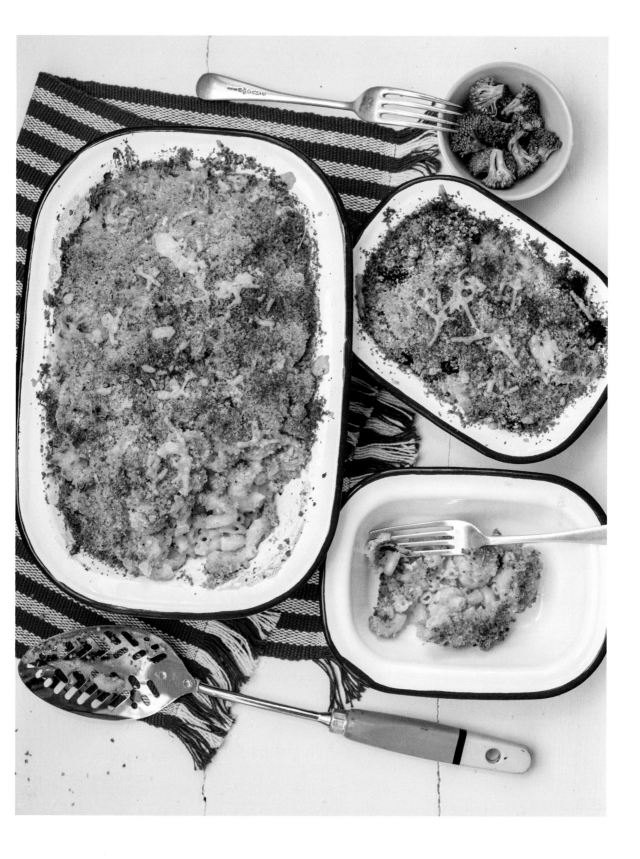

STEP 2: Melt 6 tablespoons of the butter in a large saucepan over medium-low heat and sprinkle the flour into the melted butter. Use a spatula to incorporate the flour into the butter and continue to stir the butter-flour mixture, being careful to scrape the bottom of the pan so that it doesn't become stuck. Cook this mixture for 3 to 5 minutes, until it becomes a light almond color and has a nutty aroma.

STEP 3: Warm the milk in either a microwave-safe measuring cup in the microwave or in a separate pan over low heat on the stove. It doesn't need to be boiling-hot, just warm enough to produce steam. Using the whisk continuously, mix the milk into the butter-flour mixture in a slow, steady stream. If that is difficult to manage, feel free to use a ½-cup measuring cup to work the milk into the mixture in stages. Make sure to whisk vigorously, scraping the bottom of the pan to prevent sticking and burning.

STEP 4: Raise the heat to medium-high and bring the mixture to a slow boil while stirring with the whisk to prevent lumps. Once it's bubbling, reduce the heat to medium and cook for 5 to 7 minutes to allow the flavor of the flour to cook off. Add the grated nutmeg.

STEP 5: Cut the cream cheese into ½-inch cubes and add to the saucepan, stirring until fully incorporated. Add the shredded cheese in ½-cup increments, using the spatula to stir and scrape the bottom. Finally, add the soy sauce, mustard, and salt and pepper to taste. Mix the cooked macaroni into the cheese sauce using a spatula. The reserved pasta water may be used to thin the consistency of the sauce.

STEP 6 (OPTIONAL): Preheat the oven to 375°F. Coat a casserole dish with 1 tablespoon of the butter to prevent sticking and add the cheese-covered pasta. Mix the bread crumbs, the remaining 2 tablespoons butter, the Parmesan cheese, and herbes de Provence in the bowl of a food processor. Pulse to combine. Cover the pasta with the bread crumb mixture, then cover with aluminum foil or a casserole lid. Cook in the oven for 20 minutes, or until the cheese is bubbly when you peek under the foil. Remove the foil to allow the top to brown for an additional 5 to 10 minutes, until it is golden brown to your liking. Leftovers can be stored in an airtight container refrigerated for up to 2 days, or frozen for up to 1 month.

French Fries

Fried sliced potatoes are a staple food for me. They're easy to eat and won't upset my stomach. They're not rich or heavy, and they can be adjusted spicewise depending on just how mild I need something to be.

SKILL LEVEL: EASY

COLOR: YELLOW/BROWN

KEYWORDS: SALTY, CRUNCHY, GLUTEN-FREE, VEGAN

Makes about four 4-ounce servings

1 pound starchy potatoes (like Russet)

2 tablespoons extra-virgin olive oil

Kosher salt and freshly ground black pepper to taste

1 to 2 quarts vegetable oil (optional)

EQUIPMENT

Baking sheet

Aluminum foil or parchment paper

Vegetable peeler (optional)

Chef's knife

Cutting board

Paper towels or kitchen towels

Mixing bowl

Measuring spoons

Oven mitt

Kitchen tongs

Cooling rack

Deep-fat fryer or skillet (optional)

Frying thermometer (optional)

Slotted spoon (optional)

STEP 1: Preheat the oven to 425°F. Place a rack in the center of the oven. Cover a baking sheet with aluminum foil or parchment paper to help prevent sticking and encourage browning.

STEP 2: Wash the potatoes thoroughly and either peel them or leave the skin on, according to your family's taste. Cut the potatoes into long, narrow strips, about ¼ inch thick. Use paper towels or a tea towel to dry the surface of the potatoes. They won't get crispy if they have excessive moisture. Toss the dried, cut potatoes in a large mixing bowl with the olive oil, salt, and pepper before arranging them on the baking sheet in a single layer. Give the potatoes as much space between one another as possible.

STEP 3: Bake the potatoes on the middle rack of the oven for 30 to 40 minutes, until they are browned. Using an oven mitt, remove the baking sheet from the oven and use the tongs to place the fries on a cooling rack to allow them to crisp.

STEP 4 (OPTIONAL): For particularly crunchy fries, more like fast-food or restaurant fare, cook the potatoes in the oven for only 15 to 20 minutes. Use a deep-fat fryer set to 325°F or, using a skillet with 1 inch of oil in the bottom of the pan, heat the oil over medium heat until it reaches 325°F on a frying thermometer. Cook the baked fries in the oil in batches for 2 to 3 minutes at a time, before removing with tongs or a slotted spoon and placing on a cooling rack to drain. Toss a pinch more salt and pepper on the fries.

VARIANT: Bacon and Cheese Fries

A meal unto itself, decadent and savory to the extreme. The finished fries are placed on an oven-safe cooling rack and set under the broiler for a minute to get the cheese and bacon even more melty and crispy, respectively.

COLOR: YELLOW/BROWN

KEYWORDS: TOUCHING, SALTY, HOT, GLUTEN-FREE

Makes about four 6-ounce servings

INGREDIENTS

4 strips of center-cut bacon

1 pound starchy potatoes (like Russet)

2 tablespoons extra-virgin olive oil

Kosher salt and freshly ground black pepper to taste

1 to 2 quarts vegetable oil (optional)

1½ cups shredded sharp cheddar or other tasty cheese (about 6 ounces)

RECIPE CONTINUES

EQUIPMENT

Same as above, plus:

Oven-safe cooling rack

Additional baking sheet

Step 1: Line a baking sheet with aluminum foil for easy cleanup. Place an oven-safe cooling rack on top of the baking sheet and arrange the bacon in a single row without touching. Cook in the oven as you preheat the oven to 425°F for the fries. By the time the oven is preheated, the bacon should be crispy. Remove the baking sheet with an oven mitt and set the cooked bacon aside. Drain the bacon grease for other purposes or safely discard.

Step 2: When the fries are finished to your satisfaction as per above, arrange on an oven-safe cooling rack on top of a lined baking sheet. Set the oven to Broil (top element only if using an electric stove). Sprinkle the shredded cheese on top of the fries. Place under the broiler for 1 minute. The cheese should be bubbling at this point. Using an oven mitt, remove the baking sheet from the oven. Sprinkle with the crispy bacon broken into little pieces, and put back under the broiler for 30 seconds. Remove and serve most righteously.

Sandwich Bread

A pillow. A dream. Sproingy. These are only some of the words that I would use to describe this sandwich bread. It's scarcely enriched, not even close to the degree of a brioche, yet the texture and flavor impress every time.

SKILL LEVEL: EASY

COLOR:
YELLOW/BROWN, WHITE

KEYWORDS: SOFT,
VEGETARIAN

Makes 1 large loaf (about 20 slices)

1½ cups warm (110°F) water

1 tablespoon honey or diastatic malt powder

1 tablespoon active dry yeast

3½ cups all-purpose flour, plus 1 to 2 tablespoons if the dough is particularly wet, and more flour for dusting

⅓ cup whole milk

1½ teaspoons salt

Cooking spray

1 tablespoon unsalted butter

EQUIPMENT

Measuring cups

Stand mixer with the dough hook (optional; see Making Dough by Hand—Taking a Stand Without a Mixer, page 55)

Measuring spoons

Tea towels

Small saucepan

Spatula

Cutting board or pastry board

Rolling pin

9 × 5-inch loaf pan

Small sauté pan

Pastry brush

Lame or sharp knife

Cooling rack

STEP 1: Put ½ cup of the warm water in the bowl of a stand mixer. Stir in the honey until dissolved. Sprinkle the yeast on top of the mixture, cover with a tea towel, and allow to rest in a warm, draft-free place for 5 to 10 minutes. The yeast should be foamy and bubbly.

STEP 2: While the yeast is proofing, make the tangzhong roux (see page 14) using ¼ cup of the flour and the milk.

RECIPE CONTINUES

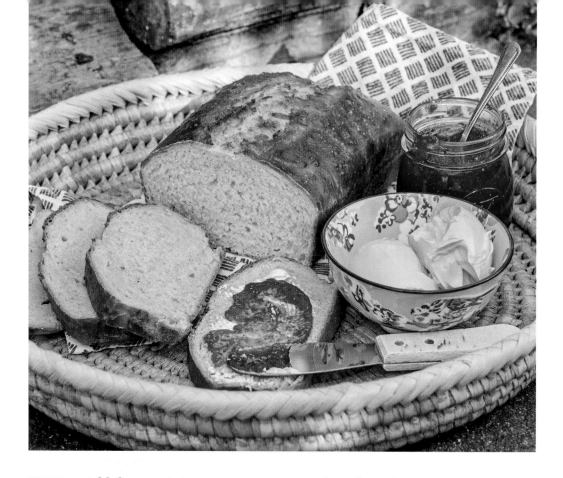

STEP 3: Add the remaining 1 cup warm water, the salt, and 1 cup of the flour to the yeast mixture. Set the stand mixer to the lowest speed, using the dough hook attachment, and mix the yeast-flour mixture into a paste. Add the remaining flour, ½ cup at a time, and give it a few moments to fully incorporate each addition. Once the additional flour has been added, add the cooled tangzhong roux and increase the speed to 2 or 3 on your mixer. Mix for 5 to 6 minutes, until the dough forms an elastic ball. The dough may still be slightly sticky or stringy due to the roux. If the dough is particularly wet, add 1 or 2 more tablespoons of flour.

STEP 4: Spray a mixing bowl with cooking spray and form the dough into a tight ball. Place it in the bowl, cover with a tea towel, and put in a warm, draft-free place until doubled in bulk. This should take 1 to 1½ hours.

STEP 5: Turn out the dough onto a cutting board or pastry board that has been lightly dusted with flour and dust a rolling pin with flour to prevent sticking. With the balls of your hands, press the dough into a rectangular shape, using the rolling pin to work out any air bubbles. After working the dough a few times, pick up the dough and turn it over, dusting it with more flour. The rectangular shape should be 1 to 1½ inches thick. Fold the dough over like a letter you are putting in an envelope. Spray a 9 × 5-inch loaf pan with cooking spray. Using your fingertips with inward pressure, tuck the sides of the dough under the shape and place the dough in the pan. Cover with a tea towel and put in a warm, draft-free place until doubled in bulk, 45 minutes to 1 hour 15 minutes.

STEP 6: Preheat the oven to 350°F. Melt the butter in a small sauté pan over low heat and brush the butter over the top of the risen dough. Use a lame or a sharp knife to cut a single vent down the center of the length of the loaf, approximately ¼ inch deep at a slight angle. Place the loaf pan in the oven and bake for 30 to 35 minutes, rotating once after 25 minutes. If you tap on the top of the loaf, there should be a hollow sound when it's done baking. After removing the loaf from the oven, give it 5 more minutes in the pan before turning it out onto a cooling rack. Allow to fully cool before slicing. Leftovers will keep for 2 to 3 days in an airtight container on the counter or up to 3 months in the freezer.

FREEZING

After the dough has been placed in the loaf pan, before the second rise, it can be frozen for later use quite readily. Place in the freezer overnight, before covering tightly with plastic wrap. To thaw, place the frozen dough in the refrigerator overnight. Set out on the counter in a warm, draft-free place, and in 3 to 4 hours it will be ready for baking.

Gluten-Free Sandwich Bread

I have a number of gluten-free friends who just wanted a sandwich. A plain sandwich. This is my answer. It's a no-fuss sandwich bread that is spongy, light, and flavorful and holds up to eating stuff between two slices of itself. The only downside is that this bread goes stale fast! So eat up, me hearties, because this loaf has got to be down in about twenty-four hours. On the bright side, you can toast and pulverize the amount you can't eat and have some nice gluten-free dried bread crumbs in stock for something special at another time.

> **SKILL LEVEL: INTERMEDIATE**
>
> **COLOR: WHITE, BROWN/YELLOW**
>
> **KEYWORDS: BREAD, SOFT, GLUTEN-FREE, VEGETARIAN**
>
> ———
>
> Makes 1 large loaf (about 20 slices)

3 cups gluten-free flour blend

2 teaspoons instant yeast

1 teaspoon salt

1½ teaspoons xanthan gum

1 cup non-skim milk, warm (100°F)

3 tablespoons honey

4 tablespoons (½ stick) unsalted butter, at room temperature

3 large eggs, at room temperature

Cooking spray

EQUIPMENT

Measuring cups

Measuring spoons

Stand mixer with the paddle attachment (optional; see Making Dough by Hand—Taking a Stand Without a Mixer, page 55)

Mixing spoon

9 × 5-inch loaf pan

Spatulas

Plastic wrap

Tea towels

Cooling rack

STEP 1: Place the flour, yeast, salt, and xanthan gum in the bowl of a stand mixer and turn on the machine to Stir.

STEP 2: Combine the warm milk and honey in a large measuring cup and stir them together until thoroughly combined. While the machine stirs the dry ingredients, slowly pour the milk-honey mixture into the flour mixture. Once all the ingredients are combined, add the butter and blend.

STEP 3: Add 1 egg to the mixture. Allow the dough to completely combine with the egg before adding the next egg. Repeat with the other 2 eggs. Increase the speed of the mixer to Medium (or 3 to 4) and allow to run for 3 minutes, until fully incorporated and the mass starts to pull away slightly from the sides of the bowl.

STEP 4: Cover the bowl with a clean tea towel and allow to rest in a warm, draft-free place for 1 hour.

STEP 5: Gently scrape down the sides of the bowl with a flexible spatula spritzed with cooking spray. Prepare a 9 × 5-inch loaf pan by spraying the inside surfaces with the cooking spray. Use the spatula to gently spoon the dough into the loaf pan, and then carefully level off the surface with the spatula. You don't want to overhandle the dough at this point, so quick and careful action is the best.

STEP 6: Spray some plastic wrap with cooking spray and cover the loaf pan, with the sprayed side of the plastic wrap down. Put the dough in a warm, draft-free place for a second rise, until it just scarcely crowns the pan. This should take 45 minutes to 1 hour. Preheat the oven to 350°F when the second rise is almost over.

STEP 7: Bake in the center of the oven on the middle rack for 40 to 45 minutes, until it's golden brown on top. Immediately remove from the oven and turn out onto a cooling rack. Allow the loaf to come to room temperature before slicing. Leftovers will stay fresh for 1 day in an airtight container on the counter or up to 3 days in the refrigerator. They can also be frozen for up to 1 month.

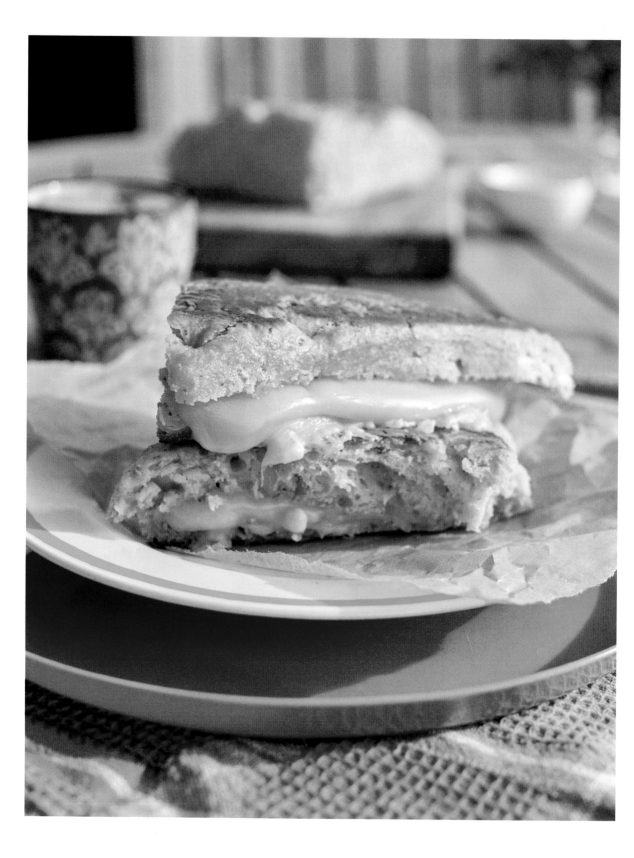

Grilled Cheese

Grilled cheese on sliced bread is the best thing since sliced bread. Explore the different cheeses of the world with this modular deliciousness-delivering platform.

SKILL LEVEL: EASY

COLOR: YELLOW/BROWN

KEYWORDS: SALTY, TOUCHING, CRUNCHY, VEGETARIAN

Makes 4 thick sandwiches

2 to 3 tablespoons whipped butter or other easily spreadable fat

8 slices of Sandwich Bread (page 113)

16 slices of Gouda or other nice melting cheese

Kosher salt and freshly ground black pepper to taste

EQUIPMENT

Large skillet or griddle

Butter knife

Spatula

STEP 1: Heat a large skillet or griddle over medium-high heat until a drop of water cast on the surface bounces off (see Tip on page 76).

STEP 2: Spread whipped butter on one side of two slices of the bread. Place four slices of the cheese on one of the unbuttered sides of the bread slices. Excessive overlap of cheese over the sides of the bread will result in a gooey mess, so do as thou wilt.

STEP 3: Put both slices of bread on the pan buttered side down and allow to toast without moving for 1 to 2 minutes, until the bread pulls away from the pan easily and is your desired degree of browned, then use a spatula to turn the slice of bread without cheese over on top of the other. Use your spatula to free the bread from the pan and turn over to the other side, cooking for 1 more minute before removing to a plate. Sprinkle with a pinch of salt and pepper. Repeat with the remaining butter, bread, and cheese.

Tomato "Robusto"

Being able to reduce this soup down to my necessary consistency was a big element to tomato soup being added to my "Will Eat" list. Pair with a classic Grilled Cheese (page 119) on a cold day and you have an oasis of calm in edible format.

SKILL LEVEL: EASY

COLOR: RED, ORANGE

KEYWORDS: SALTY, SMOOTH, VEGETARIAN, GLUTEN-FREE

Makes about ten ⅔-cup servings

2½ pounds ripe cherry tomatoes

1 large sweet onion, diced

2 celery ribs, diced

2 carrots, diced

1 tablespoon minced garlic

2 tablespoons extra-virgin olive oil

Salt and freshly ground black pepper

4 cups vegetable broth or stock

1 or 2 bay leaves

5 or 6 basil leaves

1 sprig of rosemary, destemmed

½ cup heavy cream

½ cup shredded Asiago cheese, for garnish

EQUIPMENT

Kitchen knife

Cutting board

Garlic press (optional)

Measuring spoons

Mixing bowl

Roasting pan

Measuring cups

Stockpot

Immersion blender, blender, or wire whisk

Mixing spoon

Ladle

STEP 1: Preheat the oven to 350°F. Toss the cherry tomatoes, onion, celery, carrots, garlic, and olive oil in a medium mixing bowl. Sprinkle with salt and pepper. Transfer the vegetable mixture to a large roasting pan and place in the oven on the top rack, cooking for about 30 minutes, until lightly browned on top. Turn on the broiler for 3 to 4 minutes, until the vegetables are caramelized (see Glossary, page 3).

STEP 2: Set aside the roasted vegetables. Heat the broth and 1 or 2 bay leaves in the stockpot over medium-high heat until it comes to a boil. Add the roasted vegetables and reduce the heat to medium-low. Allow to simmer, uncovered, for 15 minutes.

STEP 3: Turn off the heat, discard the bay leaves, add the basil and rosemary, and use an immersion blender until the soup reaches the desired consistency. If you do not have an immersion blender, you can wait until the soup is slightly cooler and use a standard blender. Alternatively, a wire whisk in the stockpot can help reduce the larger pieces to a more desirable size.

STEP 4: Slowly stir the heavy cream into the soup. Add salt and pepper to taste. Ladle into bowls and top each serving with 1 to 2 teaspoons of the shredded cheese. Leftovers can be stored in an airtight container in the refrigerator up to 3 days or frozen for up to 1 month. Top with more cheese when reheating.

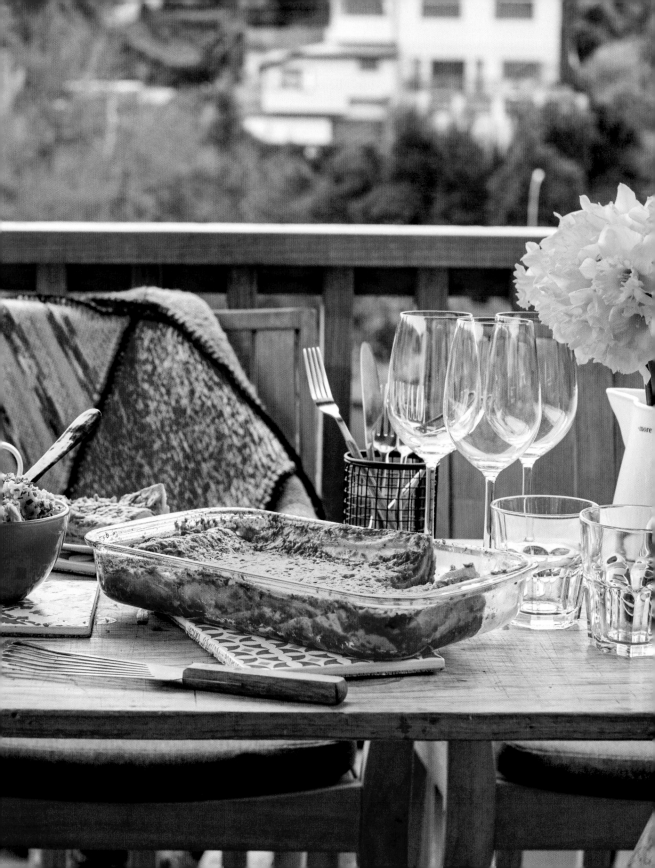

DINNER

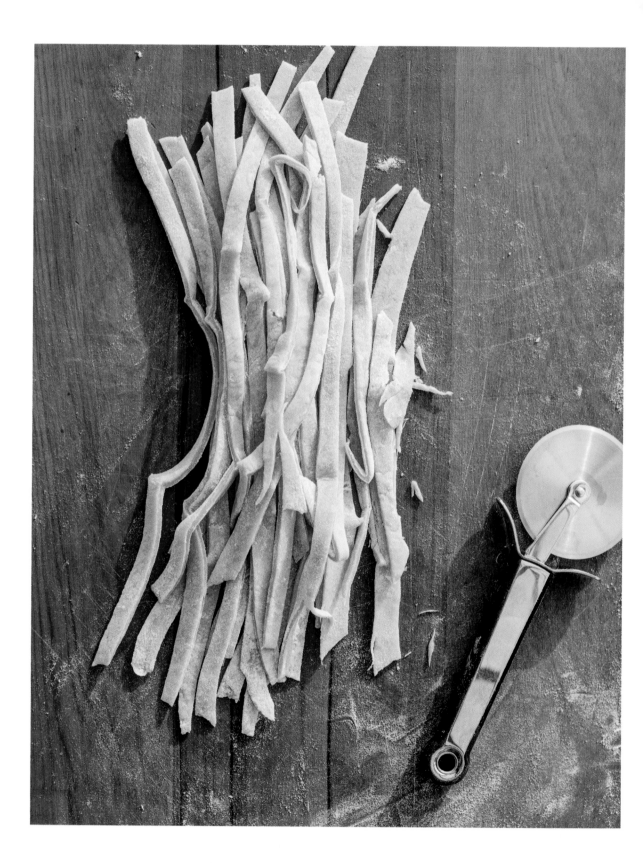

Handmade Pasta

There isn't a lot in this world that makes me happier than fresh pasta. After some practice, the process to make it becomes meditative. I gave this recipe an Intermediate difficulty in skill level, but that's just for the first and maybe second attempt. Once you get the feel of it, you'll find that making fresh pasta couldn't be any easier.

SKILL LEVEL: INTERMEDIATE

COLOR: YELLOW/BROWN

KEYWORDS: CHEWY, SALTY, VEGETARIAN

Makes four 4-ounce servings

4 extra-large eggs, plus 1 or 2 egg yolks (optional)

2¼ cups (400 g) all-purpose flour, plus 2 to 3 tablespoons for dusting

3 or 4 teaspoons kosher salt

EQUIPMENT

Mixing bowls

Kitchen thermometer

Food-safe latex-free gloves

Digital or analog kitchen scale (for precise measurements)

Measuring spoons

Fork

Plastic wrap

Pastry board

Rolling pin

Bench scraper

Knife or pasta cutter

Large stockpot

Slotted spoon or kitchen tongs

Colander

STEP 1: Set out the eggs 1 to 2 hours before you make the dough. Alternatively, put the eggs in a large bowl of 100°F water for 2 to 3 minutes.

STEP 2: Put on food-safe latex-free gloves. For simplicity's sake, place 2¼ cups (400 g) of flour in a large mixing bowl. Use your fingers or a fork to create a crater or well in the center of the flour. Crack 4 eggs into a smaller mixing bowl. If you accidentally get a piece of shell in your eggs, use a larger intact piece of shell to retrieve it. If you want a brighter, more vibrant yellow

RECIPE CONTINUES

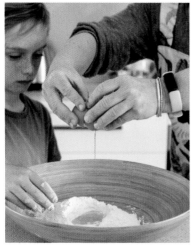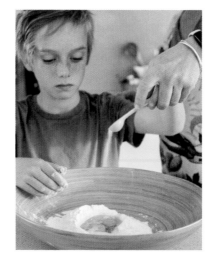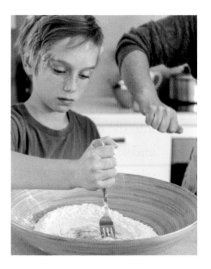
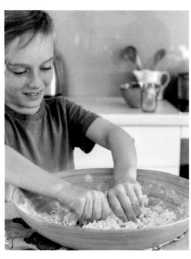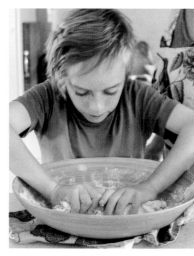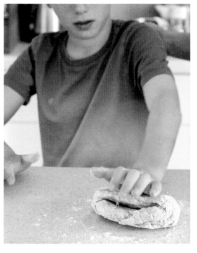
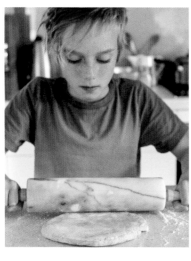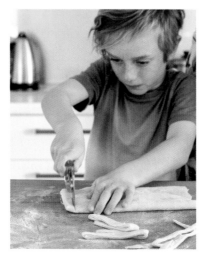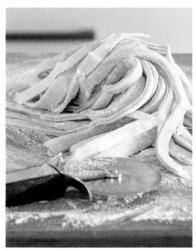

hue and richer dough, separate the yolks of 1 to 2 more eggs, if using, and add to the existing eggs.

STEP 3: Gently add the eggs to the crater in the center of the flour. Sprinkle 1 teaspoon of the salt on the eggs. Using a fork, slowly incorporate the flour into the eggs, starting with the flour closest to the eggs. Use little scooping and scraping motions, working some of the flour into the egg at a time, with the fork in the twelve o'clock position of the bowl, as you hold the bowl with your nondominant hand. Rotate the bowl, either clockwise or counterclockwise, slowly, as you incorporate the flour. Once most of the flour is worked into the eggs, use your gloved hand to press the dough into the rest of the crumbs left in the bowl, forming a ball.

STEP 4: When most of the dough is in a ball, press with the heel of your hand away from you and pull and tuck the dough back over itself. Rotate the bowl slowly as you do this. The dough will still be tough and difficult to work with. Continue to knead until the dough is smooth and elastic, like Play-Doh. Cover the dough with plastic wrap and set aside for 30 minutes. This will help to relax the gluten that has developed. Take off your gloves while you wait.

STEP 5: Put on gloves. Divide the relaxed dough into four portions. Take one of the portions and lightly sprinkle it with a little bit of flour. Sprinkle flour on a pastry board and rolling pin as well.

Cover the remaining portions with plastic wrap so they do not dry out.

Form the pasta dough into a rough rectangular shape by hand. Using the rolling pin, apply firm downward pressure away from you in the center of the dough. Pick up the dough and rotate it one quarter turn, turning it over each time. Apply more flour if it becomes sticky.

RECIPE CONTINUES

After a couple of minutes, the dough will begin to look and feel satiny. Continue to roll until you can hold the dough up to a light source and see the shadows of your fingers through the pasta sheet. Lightly dust both sides of the pasta sheet with flour and set aside, covered, while you complete the rest of the dough.

STEP 6: You can use the pasta for lasagna in whole sheets or fold a sheet loosely into thirds and use a bench scraper to provide a guide to cutting the pasta into even ribbons for fettuccine. Once cut into ribbons, use your fingers to unfold them into long sections. Sprinkle the pasta with more flour and pinch a bundle together, twirling the pasta to get a bit of flour on all the pieces so it doesn't stick. Create nests of loosely bundled pasta.

STEP 7: Fresh pasta cooks quickly. Fill a large stockpot with water and bring to a rolling boil over medium-high heat. Add 2 to 3 teaspoons of salt. Place the pasta in the boiling water for 1 to 2 minutes, until cooked to your desired doneness, using a slotted spoon or tongs to keep the pasta from bunching together. Drain in a colander.

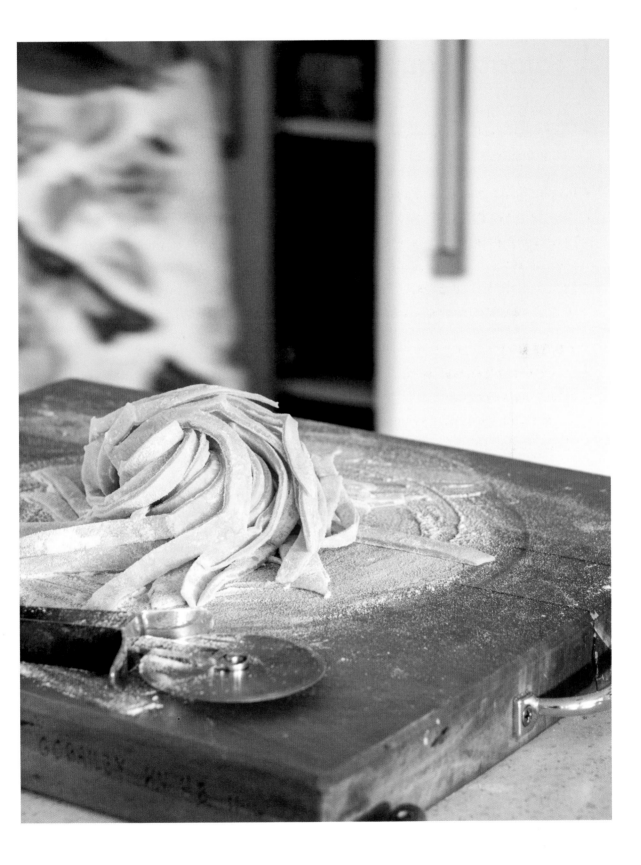

Tomato Sauce

Red sauce was such a hit-or-miss thing with me as a child. So, long story short, it turns out that I never had a problem with cooked tomato sauces. I had a problem with chunky tomato sauces. Blended and I'm in love. Chef's kiss.

SKILL LEVEL: EASY

COLOR: RED

KEYWORDS: SALTY, BITTER, HOT, SMOOTH, GLUTEN-FREE, VEGAN

Makes six ½-cup servings

¼ cup extra-virgin olive oil

2 to 3 garlic cloves, minced

1 large diced white onion

1 teaspoon kosher salt, plus more as needed

2 large carrots, diced

2 celery ribs, diced

1 (28-ounce) can Cento Peeled Tomatoes (preferred brand, but any peeled tomato works)

½ teaspoon crushed red pepper (optional)

Dried thyme, oregano, and basil to taste (optional)

Freshly ground black pepper to taste (optional)

2 cups vegetable or chicken broth

2 bay leaves

¼ teaspoon baking soda (optional)

EQUIPMENT

Measuring cups

Medium sauté pan

Garlic press (optional)

Chef's knife

Cutting board

Spatula

Blender or food processor

Measuring spoons

Large saucepan

Mixing spoon

STEP 1: Add the olive oil to a medium sauté pan over medium-low heat. When the oil shimmers, toss in the garlic and cook for about 30 seconds, until fragrant. Add the onion and a pinch of salt and cook, stirring occasionally, for 1 to 3 minutes, until translucent or lightly caramelized to taste. Next, add the carrots and celery and another pinch of salt and cook for

3 to 5 minutes, stirring occasionally. When the carrots and celery are a little browned, remove the pan from the heat.

STEP 2: Add the entire contents of the can of tomatoes to a blender and pulse until smooth. Next, add the oil-garlic-onion mixture to the blender and pulse until it's the desired texture. (If you want to turn this into a great pizza sauce, add the crushed red pepper, herbs, and salt and black pepper to taste before blending and you're done. No further steps needed.)

STEP 3: Put the vegetable mixture, broth, 1 teaspoon salt, and the bay leaves in a large saucepan over medium-high heat until it begins to bubble. Reduce the heat to low and cook, uncovered, for 30 to 40 minutes, until the sauce has reduced by half, stirring occasionally. Discard the bay leaves. Add more salt and black pepper to taste. If the sauce is too bitter for your liking, sprinkle the baking soda over the surface and stir throughout.

VARIANT: Bolognese

For Bolognese, brown 1 pound of Italian sausage or ground chuck, draining the oil before adding everything to the saucepan in Step 3.

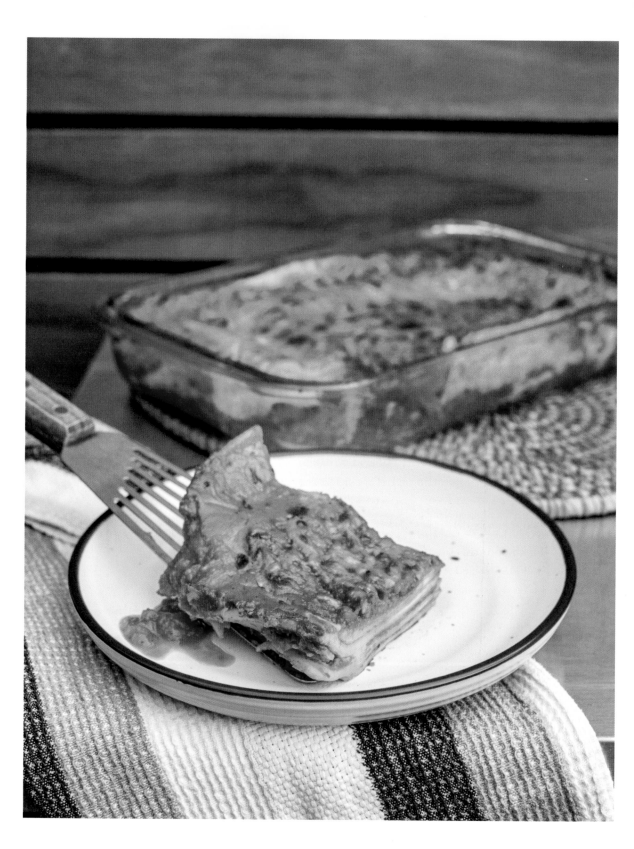

Traditional Lasagna

There is little so polarizing (foodwise!) on social media as a traditional lasagna, which utilizes a béchamel, one of the Five Mother Sauces of French cuisine. The use of cottage cheese or ricotta cheese in lasagna instead of béchamel became very popular during the '60s and '70s in the United States, for some reason.

> **SKILL LEVEL: INTERMEDIATE**
>
> **COLOR: RED, YELLOW/BROWN**
>
> **KEYWORDS: TOUCHING, SALTY, CRUNCHY, VEGETARIAN**
>
> ---
>
> Makes eight 8-ounce square wedges

BÉCHAMEL

4 tablespoons (½ stick) unsalted butter

¼ cup all-purpose flour

2 cups whole milk

1 teaspoon kosher salt, plus more as needed

Pinch of grated nutmeg

Pinch of freshly ground white or black pepper

LASAGNA

1 recipe prepared Tomato Sauce (page 130)

4 sheets of uncooked fresh pasta (Handmade Pasta, page 125, or store-bought)

Grated Parmesan or Asiago cheese

Freshly ground black pepper

Pinch of sea salt

EQUIPMENT

Medium saucepan

Measuring cups

Whisk

Small saucepan or microwave-safe measuring cup

Ladle

Mixing spoon or spatula

13 × 9-inch baking pan or any other oven-safe dish at least 1½ inches deep

Cooking spray, olive oil, or parchment paper, for the pan

Aluminum foil

Knife

RECIPE CONTINUES

STEP 1: Make the béchamel: Melt the butter in a medium saucepan over medium-low heat. Sprinkle the flour over the melted butter and whisk the combined ingredients until they are a smooth paste. Use a spatula to stir the paste continuously for 4 to 5 minutes, until the mixture begins to smell nutty and the color darkens slightly. This is called a roux in French culinary terms.

STEP 2: Warm the milk in a small saucepan or a microwave-safe cup until steaming but not a full boil, 3 to 4 minutes over medium-low heat or 1 to 2 minutes in the microwave.

STEP 3: Add the warmed milk to the roux while whisking to avoid creating clumps. It might be easier to use a ladle to spoon a smaller amount of the warmed milk into the mixture, a little at a time, than trying to hold the whole measuring cup or saucepan while whisking with the opposite hand. (See No Heroes in the Kitchen, page 59.) Once all the milk has been added, continue to stir with a spoon or spatula, carefully scraping the bottom of the pan to prevent the sauce from scalding. Add the salt to the pan. You will notice that the milk and roux begin to thicken gradually and then considerably as the heat increases. Once you get some nice bubbles and low sputters, reduce the heat to low and cook, uncovered, for 4 to 5 minutes.

You don't want the mixture to boil; simmering it will cook away the flour taste and create a more consistent product. Add a pinch more salt, the grated nutmeg, and the pepper, stirring the sauce throughout. (Optional: Traditionally, you'd use a pinch of fresh cracked white pepper to maintain the color of the dish. Black pepper works just fine by me. I'm not trying to impress anyone to this degree.) Set aside.

STEP 4: Prepare the lasagna: Preheat the oven to 400°F. Coat a 13 × 9-inch baking pan or any other oven-safe receptacle at least 1½ inches deep with some cooking spray or olive oil, or layer with parchment paper. Start by spreading one ladle of the tomato sauce evenly over the bottom of the pan. Place one of the fresh uncooked pasta sheets over the tomato sauce.

(**IMPORTANT:** Fresh pasta will expand as it cooks, so whichever size dish you are using, the pasta sheets should have 1 to 2 inches of space away from the sides. Your sheets don't need to be perfect in size and square to one another; the edges can be a little uneven, and, if anything, this unevenness just helps the folks eating your masterpiece know that you actually made it from scratch. If all the pasta sheets are touching the walls of the pan before you cook it, you might see a great escape of a little of the goodies as it all expands and runs out and over the sides.)

Put a ladle of béchamel sauce over the top of the pasta, then another ladle of tomato sauce. You don't need to be overly precise in spreading the sauces over the pasta. The process of layering in the next steps, and then cooking, will even it out.

STEP 5: Repeat the process for as many layers of pasta as you have prepared. Top the last layer with tomato sauce, some grated cheese, a few cracks of freshly ground black pepper, and a pinch of sea salt. The base pasta recipe will provide approximately four layers of pasta.

STEP 6: Place the pan in the oven for 30 to 35 minutes. Check it when it's about halfway through the cooking time, and if the top is getting overly browned, cover it with a layer of aluminum foil. Remove the pan from the oven and let rest for 10 to 15 minutes before cutting. It might be helpful to cover the pan with foil if you haven't already, to retain the moisture of the dish if you want it softer. Leave uncovered if you want it crunchier. Leftovers can be stored in an airtight container for up to 3 days in the refrigerator or up to 1 month in the freezer.

VARIANT: Deconstructed Lasagna

Some of my fellow food-averse loves out there really don't like things touching or mixed in, and a deconstructed plate for them is hardly any extra effort if you're already making the whole dish from scratch.

Makes 1 serving

INGREDIENTS
Same as above

EQUIPMENT
Pasta roller (optional)
Large pasta pot
Colander
Kitchen tongs
A divided plate (optional, but nice for presentation and honoring tastes)

STEP 1: Take the prepared béchamel, tomato sauce, and a lasagna sheet. You can also use the cut pasta surplus, especially if you had to trim the sides so it wouldn't overload the pan. Either use the excess strips or use a pasta roller to cut a few long 1-inch-wide ribbons of pasta. I like to use the crimped edge of a roller to make it a little fancier.

STEP 2: Boil 4 quarts of water in a pasta pot over medium-high heat and season the water with some salt. Drop the pasta ribbons into the boiling water and use tongs to help keep them from sticking to one another. It will cook quite quickly to al dente (2 to 3 minutes tops), but in all likelihood, if you are making a deconstructed lasagna for food aversion purposes, you might want to err on the side of cooking it until it's softer (3 to 4 minutes). Drain the pasta in a colander and add a bit of salt and pepper.

STEP 3: Twist the cooked pasta into a little bird's nest on the plate, and place some béchamel and some tomato sauce, with a good deal of real estate between them all. A divided plate is ideal. Three small ramekins, plates, or bowls might also work. (Keep an eye on the sauces before serving. If it looks like any juices are going to make a run for their dinner plate companions, it could be better to just divide them up before catastrophe strikes. An ounce of prevention and whatnot.)

VARIANT: Traditional Spinach Lasagna

Spinach is something I don't mind eating, so if I want to impress my family and friends with something that seems more "grown-up," I might make a spinach lasagna instead. It's almost identical to the traditional recipe above, but you place a layer of fresh spinach leaves, just one or two layers of leaves deep, between the béchamel and tomato sauce layers. Put a few cracks of freshly ground black pepper and sprinkle a pinch of salt on each layer of the spinach. Just make sure that there isn't any excess moisture hanging on to the spinach leaves or it could be more on the soggy side. Use a fancy salad spinner or some paper or tea towels to dry your spinach, if needed.

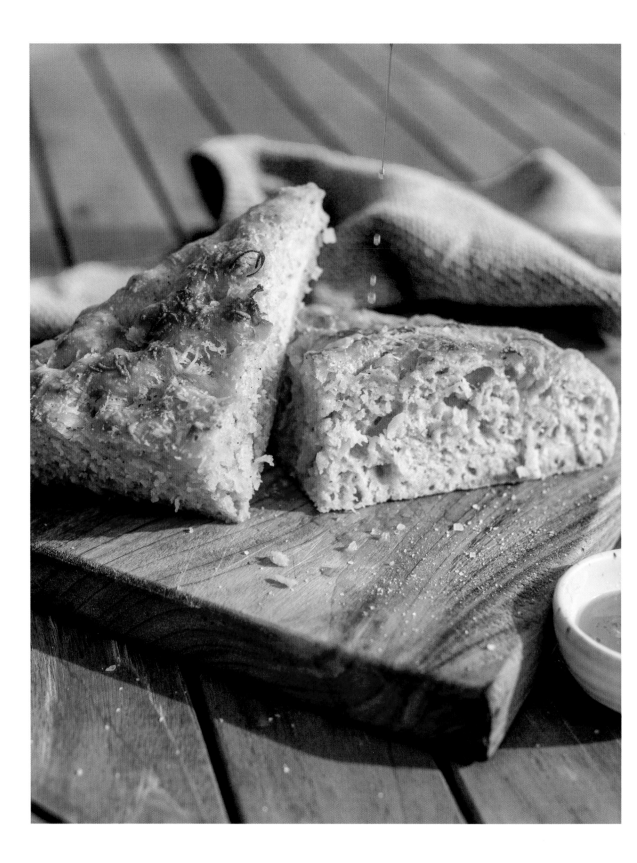

Focaccia

This is a delicious treat with infinite layers of adjustability depending on the tastes of the hungry. It can have spice, it can be herbaceous, it can be vegetable laden, or it can be a carnivore's delight. The dimpled top allows it to catch the olive oil you pour on before baking, giving it a rich coloration that tastes as good as it looks.

> **SKILL LEVEL: EASY**
>
> **COLOR: BROWN/YELLOW**
>
> **KEYWORDS: BREAD, CRUNCHY, SALTY, CHEWY, VEGAN**
>
> ---
>
> Makes sixteen 3-ounce portions

1½ cups warm (110°F to 115°F) water

1 tablespoon sulfur-free molasses

2 teaspoons kosher salt

2¼ teaspoons active dry yeast

6 cups all-purpose flour

1 teaspoon crushed red pepper

⅓ cup plus 4 tablespoons extra-virgin olive oil

1 sprig of rosemary

2 garlic cloves, crushed

EQUIPMENT

Measuring cups

Measuring spoons

Large mixing bowl

Whisk

Mixing spoons

Tea towel

9 × 9-inch baking pan

Small skillet

Small mesh strainer (optional)

Cooling rack

Cutting board

Chef's knife

STEP 1: Put the warm water, molasses, ½ teaspoon of the salt, and the yeast into a large mixing bowl and whisk thoroughly. Set aside and allow the yeast to bloom for 5 minutes in a warm, draft-free place until frothy.

STEP 2: Add the flour, 1¼ teaspoons of the salt, the crushed red pepper, and ⅓ cup of the olive oil to the bowl and stir until it has the consistency of a thick, sticky paste. Cover with a tea towel and allow to rest in a warm, draft-free place for 1 hour.

RECIPE CONTINUES

STEP 3: Spread 2 tablespoons of the olive oil in a 9 × 9-inch baking pan to coat the inner surface. Punch down the dough in the mixing bowl and pour the dough into the pan, using your fingertips to spread it out evenly.

STEP 4: Preheat the oven to 400°F. Place a rack in the center of the oven. Heat the remaining 2 tablespoons olive oil in a small skillet over medium-low heat until the oil shimmers. Sauté the rosemary and garlic in the olive oil for 30 seconds before removing from the heat. Dimple the surface of the dough with your fingertips, pressing firmly until you can feel the bottom of the pan.

Drizzle the heated olive oil over the top. Sprinkle with the remaining ¼ teaspoon salt.

OPTIONAL: Use a small mesh strainer to keep the garlic solids and rosemary leaves from being added to the baking pan.

STEP 5: Bake on the center rack of the oven for 25 to 30 minutes, until the surface is a deep golden brown. Remove from the oven and allow to cool for 5 minutes before turning out onto a cooling rack. Cut into equal portions and serve immediately. It's best consumed fresh, but will keep in an airtight container on the counter for up to 2 days or in the freezer for up to 1 month.

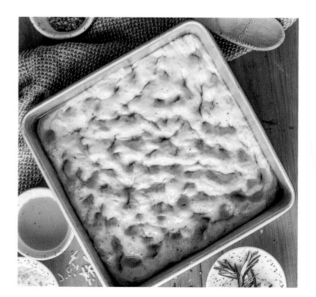

Stuffed Focaccia

This is an older-kid-friendly burger alternative. It's a little easier to eat and seems more mature for the sophisticated tween palate.

SKILL LEVEL: EASY

COLOR: YELLOW/BROWN

KEYWORDS: TOUCHING, SALTY, THICK, HOT

Makes 8 large triangular wedge sandwiches

1½ cups warm (110°F to 115°F) water

1 tablespoon honey

2¼ teaspoons active dry yeast

⅓ cup extra-virgin olive oil, plus more for oiling a large bowl

6 cups all-purpose flour, plus more for dusting

1½ teaspoons kosher salt

½ cup grated Parmesan cheese

FILLING

Safe Aromatics (per Food Preferences Profile and Safe Veggie Time-Savers, page 57)

5 tablespoons extra-virgin olive oil

1 pound bulk Italian sausage

1 sprig of rosemary

1 garlic clove, crushed

EQUIPMENT

Measuring cups

Measuring spoons

Large mixing bowl

Whisk

Mixing spoon

Large oiled mixing bowl

Medium skillet

Colander

9-inch-round cake or deep-dish pie pan

Chef's knife or pie server

STEP 1: Put the warm water, honey, and yeast in a large mixing bowl and whisk together. Allow to sit in a warm, draft-free place for 5 minutes, until frothy. Add ⅓ cup of the olive oil, along with 3 cups of the flour, the salt, and the cheese. Stir using a mixing spoon until fully incorporated. It will be a sticky ball of mess.

RECIPE CONTINUES

STEP 2: Turn the dough out onto a well-floured bench or countertop and top evenly with 1½ cups of the flour. Push and knead the flour through until it is fully combined. Do the same with the remaining 1½ cups flour until it's all incorporated. It still might be a little sticky. That's fine!

STEP 3: Put the dough in a large oiled bowl, cover, and allow to rise for 45 to 50 minutes in a warm, draft-free place. It may not double in bulk due to the density of the dough.

STEP 4: Make the filling: In a medium skillet over medium-high heat, toward the end of the rise, sauté the Safe Aromatics blend until translucent in 1 tablespoon of the olive oil. (Because these vegetables feature more prominently in the recipe, it's important that the vegetables used be according to the tastes of the hungry, following the Food Preferences Profile.) Add the bulk Italian sausage and brown the meat. Drain off the excess fat using a colander. Set aside. Retain the skillet for later.

STEP 5: Preheat the oven to 425°F. Drizzle 2 tablespoons of the olive oil into the bottom of a 9-inch-round cake pan. Divide the dough into two portions and spread one portion in the pan. Cover the dough with the cooked meat mixture. Place the second portion of dough over the top of the meat filling and spread out to cover the dish. Gingerly press straight down with your fingertips into the surface of the dough, creating little dimples that will trap some of the oil. Allow to sit. In the reserved skillet, heat the remaining 2 tablespoons olive oil over medium-high heat. Place the rosemary and garlic into the oil and heat for 30 seconds. Remove the pan from the heat and discard the rosemary and garlic. Drizzle the fragrant, hot oil over the top of the dough.

STEP 6: Place the pan in the oven for 25 to 30 minutes, until the top is golden brown. Take out of the oven and allow to cool for 5 minutes before removing from the pan. Allow to cool for another 5 minutes before cutting into wedges.

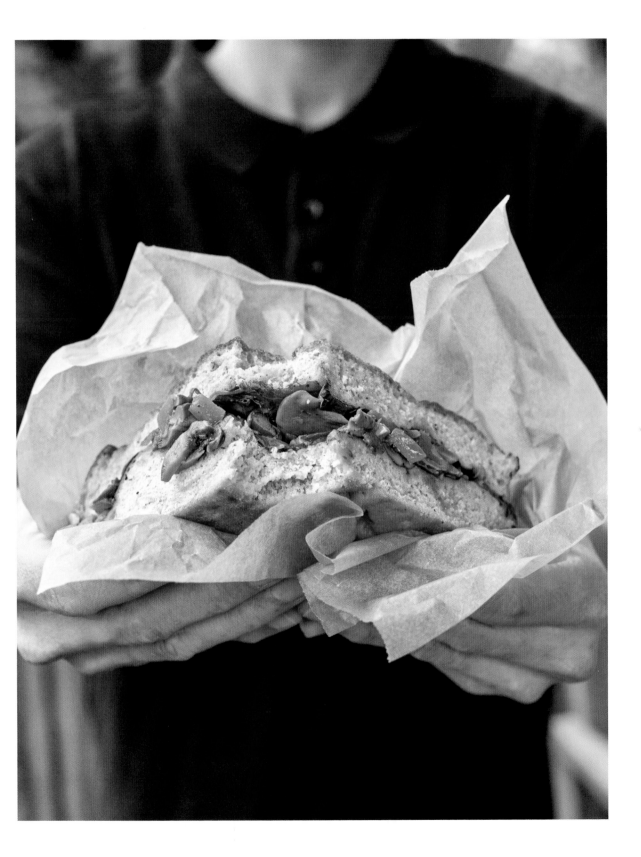

VARIANT: Vegan Stuffed Focaccia

I have heard rave reviews of this dish, which I created for the cookbook in your hands! As almost everything I am averse to exists in this meal, I can attest that each individual component is probably delicious . . .

COLOR: RED, YELLOW/BROWN, GREEN

Makes 8 large portions

INGREDIENTS

Same as above, with no meat or
  cheese, plus:

2 tablespoons extra-virgin olive oil

1 to 2 large garlic cloves, minced

1 large sweet onion, diced

2 celery ribs, diced

1 large carrot, diced

Salt and freshly ground
  black pepper

1 sprig of rosemary, destemmed

2 parsnips, peeled and sliced

1 cup cherry tomatoes, halved

1 tablespoon balsamic vinegar

2 cups button mushrooms, sliced

2 cups fresh spinach

EQUIPMENT

Same as above

Step 1: Prepare the dough as above. For the filling, heat a medium skillet with the olive oil over medium heat. Sauté the garlic, onion, celery, and carrot until browned, 7 to 8 minutes, stirring occasionally. Add a pinch of salt and pepper at the start and end of the process.

Step 2: Add half of the destemmed rosemary along with the parsnips, cherry tomatoes, and balsamic vinegar, stirring occasionally, and cook, covered, for 5 to 7 minutes, until the parsnips start to soften. Add a pinch of salt and pepper at the start and finish of this step.

Step 3: Add the sliced mushrooms and remainder of the destemmed rosemary, with a pinch of salt and pepper. Toss the mushrooms and coat them in the pan juices. Cook, uncovered, for 1 to 2 minutes, until fragrant and most of the juices have cooked off, stirring constantly—be careful not to break up the mushrooms.

Step 4: Follow the process of the Stuffed Focaccia. Put half of the fresh spinach leaves on either side of the filling between the two layers of dough, cooking as described above.

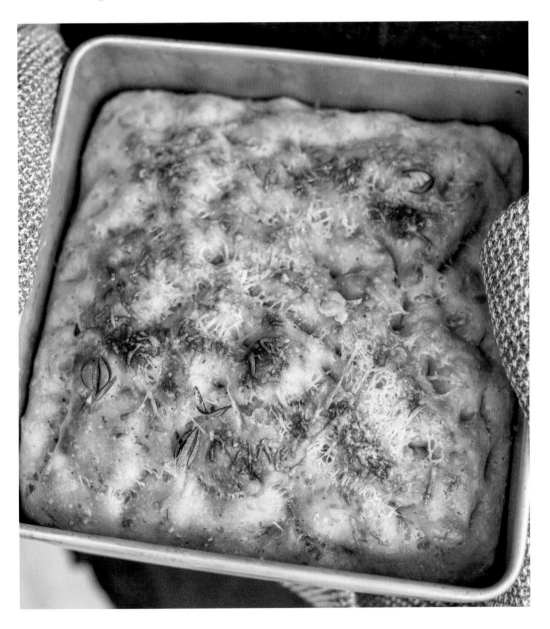

The Ultimate Fowl Champion

Spatchcock is one of my favorite words of all time. It's even fun to say. What is it, you may ask? It's the process of removing the spine of a bird like a predatory alien in a classic action movie and breaking the breastbone with solid force so that the bird is flat. Spatchcocking is the easiest way to ensure that your poultry will cook evenly, stay moist, and take a fraction of the time to cook. Case in point: Many people think that turkey is just bad, but that's because they've never had it prepared properly. With some preparation, you can make a turkey that has succulent, flavorful white meat and blow the minds of people who have preconceived notions about what turkey tastes like. Even a simple chicken roasted with the spatchcock method becomes a hero, and that's why I call this the Ultimate Fowl Champion.

SKILL LEVEL: INTERMEDIATE (IF SPATCHCOCKING IT YOURSELF); EASY (IF YOUR FRIENDLY NEIGHBORHOOD BUTCHER IS)

COLOR: YELLOW/BROWN, WHITE

KEYWORDS: HOT, STRINGY, SALTY, CHEWY

Makes 2 to 3 servings per (uncooked) pound

1 (12- to 14-pound) turkey or (5- to 6-pound) chicken

Kosher salt and freshly ground black pepper (see Note)

EQUIPMENT

Strong kitchen shears

Paring knife (optional)

Paper towels

Oven-safe wire rack

Full baking sheet (or half sheet for chicken)

Plastic wrap

Meat thermometer

Aluminum foil

Chef's knife

Carving board

STEP 1: Either have a butcher spatchcock a turkey or do it as follows: **Make sure your bird is completely thawed.** If it's even slightly frozen, it's going to turn an already difficult task into a Herculean one. Turn the turkey breast side down. Take a pair of strong kitchen shears and cut along either side of the backbone, which is right in the middle of the subject when the breast side is down. The backbone is 1 to 2 inches wide, and you want to start with the larger cavity of the bird pointed toward you. It's going to take some hand strength. Start at the cavity and work along one side until you cut completely down that side. (If you encounter some resistance, you might need to move your shears over slightly, away from the center, because you might be catching a vertebra.) Then do the other side along the spine.

STEP 2: After you've removed the backbone, you can hoist it to the sky and give a battle cry. Or not. I'm not the kitchen police. Turn the bird back over, breast side up, and spread open the butterflied poultry so that when you apply downward force and break the breastbone, it lies flat. Unfortunately, this will also break the wishbone. You can remove the wishbone prior to this step if you so desire: With your fingers, explore the neck cavity of the bird pointed toward you. You might need to use a paring knife to help cut away some of the skin and expose the area to probing. The bone is less than an inch below the flesh and it frames either side of the neck cavity. To help your visualization, those are the pieces that you grasp when you pull against your cousin contender and see if the gods favor you in your wish of supremacy.

You should be able to feel the two bony prongs and use your knife to slice horizontally under and along either side of the knobs. Scrape behind those bones in the pocket you just created with the tip of the knife pointed up toward the center of the "V" and free it. It's much more complicated-sounding than it is, and once you've done it a couple of times, it's a breeze. If you're struggling, there are a number of videos of the process online.

RECIPE CONTINUES

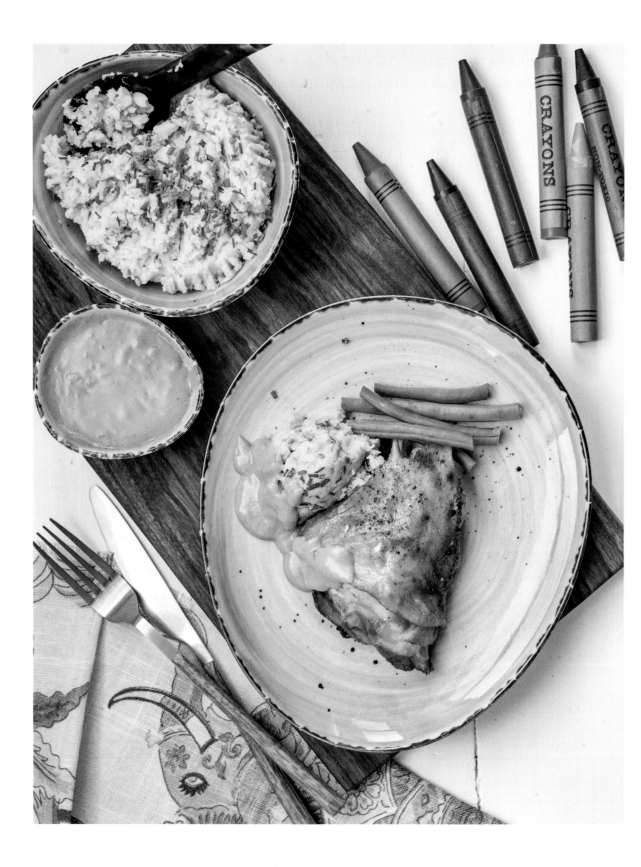

Removing the wishbone isn't just a matter of keeping the ancient rituals; it also helps you carve the bird more cleanly when it's prepared.

STEP 3: Dry the skin of the bird with some paper towels and place it breast side up on a wire rack over a baking sheet. Aggressively sprinkle salt and pepper over the entire surface of the bird. You want to be able to see the salt on the bird, but you don't want to encrust the bird in salt. This seemingly elusive balance can be achieved by aiming for about ½ teaspoon of kosher salt per pound of meat. Wrap the entire thing in plastic and set it in the fridge.

We are dry brining, my friend.

Depending on the weight of the bird, this can take anywhere from several hours to a couple of days. A big ole turkey will take at least 2 days—a full 24 hours with the bird covered in plastic wrap and another 12 uncovered in the fridge. After you take the plastic wrap off the bird, you may be worried about pathogens. As long as there aren't standing bird juices on the sheet (just drain them if there are), the salt will combat any bacteria, like a tiny sodium shield. Salt preservation of meats is a big reason we survived as a species, and you'll be cooking this bird soon enough, so fret not.

An average-size whole chicken can be readily dry brined in 4 hours covered and 1 hour uncovered. Duck takes a little longer due to the fattiness of the breast, and you want a much drier skin.

STEP 4: Preheat the oven to 450°F. I like to throw a peeled, quartered onion, a few clean celery ribs, a carrot broken in two, and a smashed garlic clove on the surface of the baking sheet, along with any fresh herbs I've got lying around. Pour a little water into the bottom of the baking sheet to prevent excessive smoking. Cook at 450°F for 15 minutes. Reduce the temperature to 400°F for the remainder of the cook time.

RECIPE CONTINUES

A 12-pound spatchcocked, dry-brined turkey only takes about 45 minutes total.

An average chicken takes about 25 minutes.

(Yes, you read that right.)

You'll want a meat thermometer stuck in the thickest part of the meat (the thigh) to register 165°F. When that target is reached, pull that beauty out.

Tent with foil for 15 minutes before carving.

NOTE

Kosher salt is important. The granules of typical iodized table salt are too small. They will permeate the meat too quickly and thus rapidly oversalt the product. If you can't find kosher salt, use some coarse-ground salt—just avoid table salt or iodized salt.

Pan-Fried Salmon Fritters

My grandmother made salmon patties for me and her family growing up, and I loved them so much. They were the only kind of fish I would eat with a recognizable name (hint: fish sticks don't count). She made a version with saltine crackers, and while I wouldn't turn a dish made with her recipe away, I've created my own that I make as an homage to my dearly departed gramma. It remains a kitchen staple.

Don't turn your nose up at the prepackaged cooked salmon (without bones or skin) until you've tried this. Once in a while one of my cousins will ask for this recipe, longing for a taste of the past. Please accept this, dear readers, as a time capsule of my childhood, and so I can tell those relatives that they need to buy my cookbook if they want to know it. Great Glob, why haven't they bought it already?

SKILL LEVEL: EASY

COLOR: YELLOW/BROWN, WHITE

KEYWORDS: SALTY, CRUNCHY, HOT

Makes six 4- to 5-ounce fritters

2 (6-ounce) pouches cooked salmon in water (deboned, no skin)

2 large eggs, at room temperature

1 teaspoon kosher salt, plus more to taste

1 teaspoon low-sodium soy sauce

1 teaspoon Dijon mustard

¼ teaspoon crushed red pepper

2 garlic cloves, minced

1 cup dried bread crumbs

½ cup grated Parmesan cheese

3 tablespoons extra-virgin olive oil, for frying

Freshly ground black pepper to taste

RECIPE CONTINUES

EQUIPMENT

Mixing bowls

Fork

Measuring spoons

Whisk

Measuring cups

Plastic wrap

Latex-free disposable gloves (optional)

Cookie dough or ice cream scoop (optional)

Parchment paper

Medium skillet

Spatula

Cooling rack

STEP 1: Empty the contents of the salmon pouches into a medium mixing bowl and flake with a fork. In a separate small bowl, combine the eggs, salt, soy sauce, mustard, crushed red pepper, and garlic. Whisk the mixture until it comes together.

STEP 2: Add the bread crumbs and cheese to the salmon and use a fork to combine thoroughly. The mixture will be very crumbly and dry.

Pour the egg mixture over the salmon mixture and use a fork to combine until it can hold together with pressure. **NOTE:** It's very possible to overwork the salmon fritter as soon as you add the egg. It will be quite dry, and deft maneuvers are recommended. You don't want the mixture to be stuck together with the density of a hockey puck, more like wet sand before you build a sandcastle.

Cover the bowl with plastic wrap and put it in the fridge for at least 30 minutes.

STEP 3: Remove the bowl from the fridge and divide the contents into six equal portions, formed into balls, 4 to 5 ounces in size. This can be done with disposable gloves, if using, to keep from having to touch the food (my preference). It can also be done using an ice cream scoop or measured cookie dough scoop to ensure even portions and make quick work of the task. Once the contents are measured out, form them into hockey puck–like shapes that are the same size and thickness so they cook at the same rate.

NOTE: You don't want the fritters to be more than 1 inch thick or they will take too long to cook.

Set aside the prepared fritters on a piece of parchment paper.

STEP 4: Preheat the oil in a medium skillet over medium-high heat until it shimmers. Gingerly place as many fritters as can fit in the pan with ample space between them, being careful not to overcrowd the pan (you don't want the temperature of the oil to drop). When you first place the fritters in the pan, use a spatula to apply a little pressure and flatten them out a bit, but not so much pressure as to cause the fritters to crack along the sides. Hit with a bit of salt and pepper. Cook, untouched, for 4 minutes.

STEP 5: If you shake the pan a bit and the fritters move freely without sticking, use the spatula to turn them over. Otherwise give them a bit more time, until they move freely.

When turned over, add a bit more salt and pepper, apply just a touch of pressure to the tops with the spatula as before, and cook for 3 minutes, undisturbed, before jiggling the pan a bit to see if they have developed a crust.

Use your spatula to peek at the bottom of the fritters, and if they are a golden brown, remove them from the pan and place them on a cooling rack, freshest cooked side down. Sprinkle with a pinch more salt and pepper. Cool for 5 minutes before serving. Leftovers will keep in an airtight container in the refrigerator for up to 3 days or in the freezer for up to 1 month.

Chili with Beans

I love a good kitchen staple meal. Boasting a humble provenance from an aromatic bag chilling in the freezer and some inexpensive-to-keep-on-hand canned goods, this chili is a phenom. You can use a chili seasoning blend you already like, but I'm particularly partial to mine. The base provided is a simple yet hearty vegan dish where the meat won't be missed. The spice level is variable to the needs of the hungry. The consistency is also extremely modular. I can attest that if you follow the instructions, there won't be a crunchy or squishy bit to distract the food averse. However, you can take some extra precautions and blend the aromatics until smooth and/or blend the diced tomatoes prior to adding them to the dish.

SKILL LEVEL: EASY

COLOR: RED, YELLOW/ BROWN, GREEN

KEYWORDS: TOUCHING, MIXED IN, SALTY, THICK, SPICY

Makes about twelve ⅔-cup servings

1 (1-pound) bag of dried kidney beans or 3 (15-ounce) cans red kidney beans, undrained

3 tablespoons extra-virgin olive oil

2 bay leaves

2 celery ribs, diced

2 large sweet onions,

1 whole and peeled and 1 diced

4 garlic cloves, minced

3 carrots, 1 broken into a few pieces and 2 diced

2 teaspoons salt, plus more as needed

1 (6- to 8-ounce) can chipotle peppers in

adobo sauce, diced (if a less spicy chili is desired, only use the peppers, rinsed of excess sauce and diced small)

3 tablespoons mild chili powder

1 tablespoon ground cumin

1 to 2 teaspoons cayenne pepper

2 teaspoons smoked paprika

1 teaspoon freshly ground black pepper

¼ to ½ teaspoon crushed red pepper

1 teaspoon dark brown sugar

1 teaspoon onion powder

1 teaspoon garlic powder

1 teaspoon dried oregano

1 teaspoon ground mustard

Pinch of grated nutmeg

Pinch of ground ginger

Pinch of allspice

Pinch of ground cinnamon

2 cups vegetable broth

2 (15-ounce) cans diced tomatoes, juice and all

2 (15-ounce) cans tomato sauce

2 to 3 jalapeño peppers, diced (optional)

1 (6- to 8-ounce) can mild green chiles

1 tablespoon low-sodium soy sauce

1 (15-ounce) can vegan refried beans

Shredded cheese, sour cream, or cooked rice for accompaniment (optional)

EQUIPMENT

Large stockpot

Measuring spoons

Chef's knife

Cutting board

Colander

Bowl

Mixing spoon or spatula

Measuring cups

Disposable latex-free gloves (for handling the peppers)

Food processor, immersion blender, or standard blender

STEP 0 (OPTIONAL): Bring the dried kidney beans to a simmer over medium-high heat in a large stockpot with enough salted water to cover them by 2 inches. Add 1 tablespoon of the olive oil. Reduce the heat to low. Throw in 1 bay leaf, 1 diced celery rib, the peeled whole onion, 2 minced garlic cloves, and 1 carrot broken into a few pieces to flavor the beans as they cook and make your house smell edible. No need to soak the beans. Just throw everything in the pot. Don't worry about the veggies being sautéed or diced if they are clean. Cook for about 2 hours, partially covered, so some steam can escape. Check every 30 minutes to make sure there is enough water to submerge the beans while cooking. When the beans are fork-tender, remove the stockpot from the heat and drain the beans using a colander over a bowl or other receptacle. Pull out and discard the smooshed veggies and

RECIPE CONTINUES

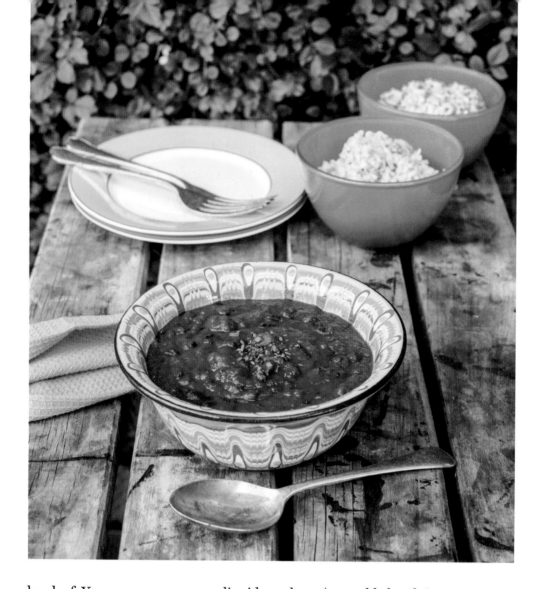

bay leaf. You can use any excess liquid as a bean/vegetable broth in Step 2. Reserve the beans. They freeze great in a gallon-size zip-top plastic bag. I make a few batches at a time to have these sachets of deliciousness on hand.

STEP 1: Heat the remaining 2 tablespoons olive oil in the stockpot over medium-high heat. Add the remaining 2 minced garlic cloves and stir for 30 seconds before adding the diced onion and a pinch of salt. Stir frequently for 1 to 2 minutes, until the onion is translucent. Add the remaining celery rib and the 2 remaining carrots along with a pinch of salt and cook until the onion takes on a light brown color, stirring occasionally. This should take 4 to 5 more minutes.

STEP 2: Add the diced chipotle peppers to the aromatics in the pot. Include the sauce for a spicier end product. Incorporate the chili powder, cumin, cayenne, paprika, salt, black pepper, crushed red pepper, brown sugar, onion powder, garlic powder, dried oregano, ground mustard, nutmeg, ground ginger, allspice, and cinnamon. Stir and cook in the pot for 1 to 2 minutes before adding the vegetable broth. At this point, you need to decide if you want the aromatics blended or not. If you do, pull the pot from the heat and run the slightly cooled mixture through a standard blender or food processor until smooth, or use an immersion blender. If pulled from the heating element to blend smooth, reheat the puree over medium-high heat.

STEP 3: Either puree the diced tomatoes in a blender or in the pot with the aromatics if so desired, or add both the diced tomatoes and the tomato sauce to the pot, along with the remaining bay leaf. This is also a good time to decide if you'll be adding the optional jalapeños and if you'll be blending them. Add the canned mild green chiles, soy sauce, and kidney beans (either from the beans you made in Step 0, or straight from the can, with juices and all). Cook, uncovered, for 25 to 30 minutes over low heat, stirring occasionally, until the beans start to release their starch and become sticky. Discard the bay leaf.

STEP 4: Four to 5 minutes before serving, add the can of refried beans a few large spoonfuls at a time, squishing the beans against the side of the pot and then stirring throughout the chili. It will add a density and heartiness to the dish. Serve in a bowl with some favored toppings, or over some cooked rice. Leftovers can be stored in an airtight container in the refrigerator for up to 3 days or in the freezer for up to 1 month.

VARIANT: My Chili con Carne

This is literally what it says it is "on the tin": chili with meat. And beans.

NOTE: I refuse to argue about whether beans should be in chili. That's why I call this recipe My Chili con Carne. No arguments. Says right there beans are in the chili.

INGREDIENTS

Same as above, minus the refried beans, plus:

1½ pounds ground chuck beef

1 teaspoon extra-virgin olive oil

EQUIPMENT

Same as above

Step 0 (**Optional**): Bring the dried kidney beans to a simmer over medium-high heat in a large stockpot with enough salted water to cover them by 2 inches. Add 1 tablespoon of the olive oil. Reduce the heat to low. Throw in 1 bay leaf, 1 diced celery rib, the peeled whole onion, 2 minced garlic cloves, and 1 carrot broken into a few pieces to flavor the beans as they cook and make your house smell edible. No need to soak the beans. Just throw everything in the pot. Don't worry about the veggies being sautéed or diced if they are clean. Cook for about 2 hours, partially covered, so some steam can escape. Check every 30 minutes to make sure there is enough water for the beans to remain submerged while cooking. When the beans are fork-tender, remove the stockpot from the heat and drain the beans using a colander over a bowl or other receptacle. Pull out and discard the smooshed veggies and bay leaf. You can use any excess liquid as a bean/vegetable broth in Step 2. Reserve the beans. They freeze great in a gallon-size zip-top plastic bag. I make a few batches at a time to have these sachets of deliciousness on hand.

Step 1: Brown the ground beef in the 1 teaspoon olive oil in the stockpot over medium-high heat. Break it into smaller pieces with a mixing spoon.

Add a pinch of salt and pepper at the start and finish of the process. Drain the excess fat with a colander before setting the beef aside.

Step 2: Heat the remaining 2 tablespoons olive oil in the stockpot over medium-high heat. Add the remaining 2 minced garlic cloves and stir for 30 seconds before adding the diced onion and a pinch of salt. Stir frequently for 1 to 2 minutes, until the onion is translucent. Add the remaining celery rib and the 2 remaining carrots along with a pinch of salt and cook until the onion takes on a light brown color, stirring occasionally. This should take 4 to 5 more minutes.

Step 2: Add the diced chipotle peppers to the aromatics in the pot. Include the sauce for a spicier end product. Incorporate the chili powder, cumin, cayenne, paprika, 2 teaspoons of salt, the black pepper, crushed red pepper, brown sugar, onion powder, garlic powder, dried oregano, ground mustard, nutmeg, ground ginger, allspice, and cinnamon. Stir and cook in the pot for 1 to 2 minutes before adding the vegetable broth. At this point, you need to decide if you want the aromatics blended or not. If you do, pull the pot from the heat and run the slightly cooled mixture through a standard blender or food processor until smooth, or use an immersion blender. If pulled from the heating element to blend smooth, reheat the puree over medium-high heat.

Step 3: Either puree the diced tomatoes in a blender or in the pot with the aromatics if so desired, or add both the diced tomatoes and the tomato sauce to the pot, along with the remaining bay leaf. This is also a good time to decide if you'll be adding the optional jalapeños and if you'll be blending them. Add the canned mild green chiles, soy sauce, cooked ground beef, and kidney beans (either from the beans you made in Step 0, or straight from the can, with juices and all). Cook, uncovered, for 25 to 30 minutes over low heat, stirring occasionally, until the beans start to release their starch and become sticky. Discard the bay leaf. Serve in a bowl with your favored toppings, or over some cooked rice. Leftovers are exceptionally delicious, as the flavors have more time to meld, and can be stored in an airtight container in the refrigerator for up to 3 days or in the freezer for up to 1 month.

Lentil Soup

I prefer my lentils with a bit of bite to them. I don't want a big mouth of mush, as that's too close to baby food for my liking. This is a tried-and-true recipe for tasty, rib-sticking grub.

SKILL LEVEL: EASY

COLOR: RED, ORANGE, YELLOW/BROWN, GREEN

KEYWORDS: HOT, THICK, SALTY, VEGAN, GLUTEN-FREE

Makes about eight ⅔-cup servings

2 tablespoons extra-virgin olive oil

2 garlic cloves, minced

1 large white onion, diced

2 celery ribs, diced

2 large carrots, diced

1 teaspoon kosher salt, plus more to taste

1 orange bell pepper, cored, seeded, and diced

2 (15-ounce) cans diced tomatoes, juice and all

4 cups vegetable stock

2 bay leaves

1 teaspoon smoked paprika

1 teaspoon ground cumin

¼ cup fresh lemon juice (about 1 lemon)

2 teaspoons low-sodium soy sauce

8 ounces dried lentils

Freshly ground black pepper

EQUIPMENT

Measuring spoons

Large stockpot

Mixing spoon

Chopping board

Chef's knife

Measuring cups

Immersion blender (optional)

STEP 1: Heat the olive oil in the stockpot over medium heat until it shimmers. Sauté the garlic for 30 seconds, stirring frequently. Add the onion and cook for 2 minutes, before adding the celery and carrots and cooking for 2 more minutes. Add a pinch of salt. Add the bell pepper, canned diced tomatoes, and vegetable stock.

STEP 2: Bring the contents to a simmer over medium heat and cook, uncovered, for 5 minutes. If a smoother consistency is desired, use the optional immersion blender at this point. Add the bay leaves, paprika, cumin, lemon juice, soy sauce, 1 teaspoon salt, and lentils. Reduce the heat to medium-low and cook, covered, while allowing a little steam to escape. Cook for 30 to 45 minutes, until the lentils are the desired tenderness. Discard the bay leaves and hit with salt and pepper to taste before serving. Leftovers can be stored in an airtight container in the refrigerator for up to 3 days or in the freezer for up to 1 month.

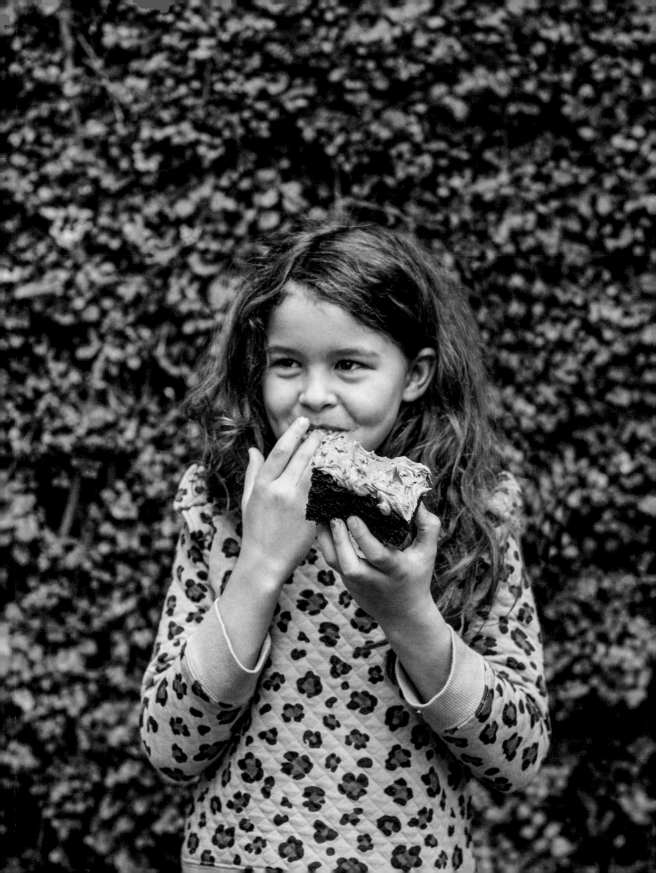

TREATS

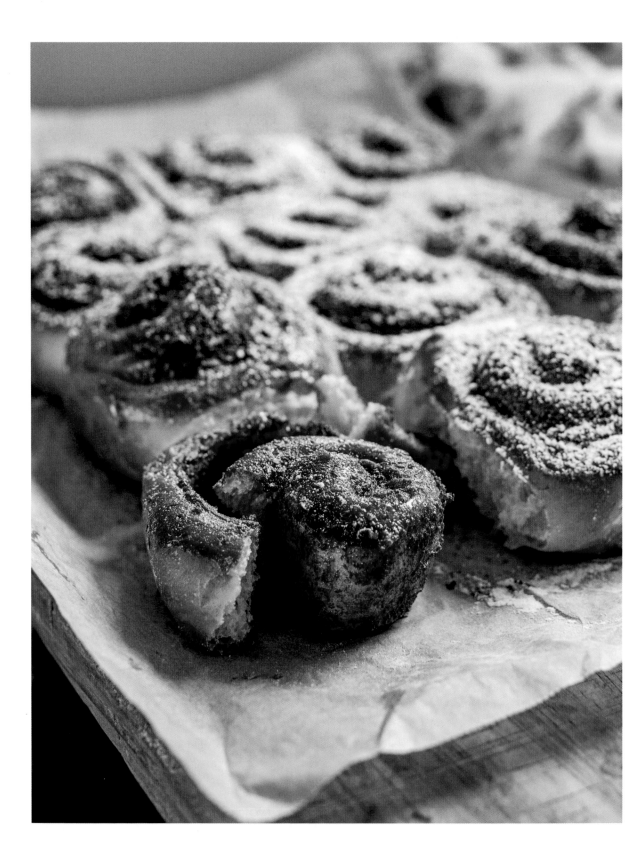

Signature Cinnamon Scrolls

These cinnamon rolls are a game changer. I've spent almost two decades perfecting this recipe, with dozens of iterations, and it is perhaps my favorite culinary feat. If I were a betting enby, I'd put money down that after a little practice, these cinnamon loves would stand toe to toe with any other out there—and even come out ahead.

> SKILL LEVEL:
> INTERMEDIATE
>
> COLOR: YELLOW/BROWN, WHITE
>
> KEYWORDS: SOFT, SWEET, VEGETARIAN
>
> ———
>
> Makes 12 large rolls

DOUGH

½ cup warm (100°F) whole milk

½ cup warm (100°F) water

¼ cup honey

2¼ teaspoons active dry yeast

1 large egg

1 teaspoon kosher salt

2 tablespoons fresh orange juice

3¼ to 3¾ cups whole wheat flour, plus more for dusting the rolling pin and the rolling surface

⅓ cup whole milk

Cooking spray

FILLING

1 large egg, lightly beaten

⅔ cup light brown sugar, plus more for the bottom of the baking pan

2 tablespoons ground cinnamon

Pinch of grated nutmeg

1 tablespoon unsalted butter, melted, for brushing

Vanilla Cream Cheese Buttercream Frosting (page 171)

EQUIPMENT

Measuring cups

Stand mixer with the dough hook (optional; see Making Dough by Hand—Taking a Stand Without a Mixer, page 55)

Measuring spoons

Small saucepan

Spatula

Mixing bowls

Kitchen towels

Rolling pin

Whisk

Pastry brush

Fork

13 × 9-inch baking pan

Parchment paper

Kitchen knife

RECIPE CONTINUES

STEP 1: Add the warm milk, warm water, and honey to the bowl of a stand mixer. Sprinkle the yeast on top and allow to bloom for 5 minutes, until frothy.

STEP 2: Add the egg, salt, and orange juice to the bowl and combine using a dough hook. Set it to Stir or the lowest setting. Add 2 cups of the flour and allow it to incorporate for 2 to 3 minutes.

STEP 3: Make a tangzhong roux (see page 14) using the ⅓ cup milk and ¼ cup of the flour. Add the roux to the stand mixer and increase the speed of the mixer to 3 or Medium-Low. Add the remaining flour in ½-cup increments, allowing the flour to fully incorporate. Stop adding flour when the dough starts to pull a little from the sides of the bowl. Knead for 7 to 9 minutes. The dough should be smooth and elastic, and slightly sticky to the touch.

STEP 4: Spray a large bowl with cooking spray. Put the dough into the bowl, cover with a kitchen towel, and allow it to rise in a warm, draft-free place for 1½ to 2 hours, until doubled in bulk.

STEP 5: Punch down the dough and roll the dough out with a floured rolling pin on a lightly floured surface into a rectangle about the size of a 13 × 9-inch baking pan.

STEP 6: Make the filling: Whisk the egg in a small bowl with 1 tablespoon of cool water. Mix the brown sugar, cinnamon, and nutmeg in a separate small bowl.

STEP 7: Brush the rolled-out dough with the egg wash and coat evenly. Sprinkle the sugar mixture on the egg-washed dough. Use a fork to press the mixture into the dough. Roll the dough along the long side into a log, pressing down lightly as you go, pinching the dough sealed.

STEP 8: Put the parchment paper into the bottom of a 13 × 9-inch baking pan. Spray it with cooking spray and sprinkle a bit of brown sugar on the parchment paper. Cut the dough into 14 evenly sized sections, discarding the end pieces. Place the rolls in the pan, a few inches apart.

STEP 9: Cover the pan with a kitchen towel and allow to rise in a warm, draft-free place for 30 minutes, or until doubled in bulk.

RECIPE CONTINUES

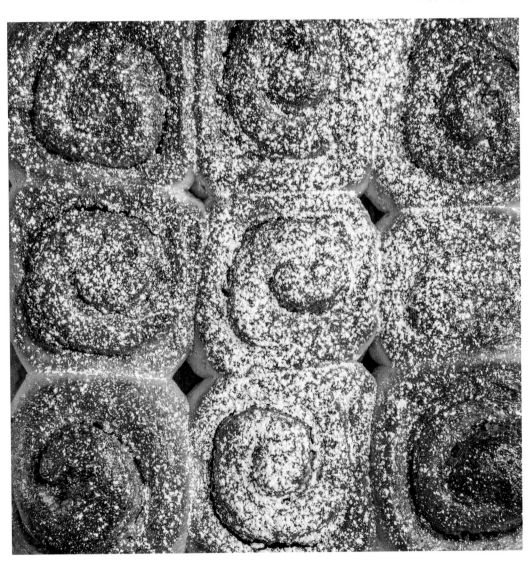

STEP 10: Preheat the oven to 350°F. Brush the tops of the rolls with the melted butter and place on the middle rack of the oven. Bake for 15 minutes. Rotate the pan to allow it to bake evenly and bake for another 15 minutes, or until golden brown and delicious.

STEP 11: Remove the cinnamon rolls from the oven and allow to cool to room temperature before frosting. Leftovers will keep, tightly covered in the pan, in the refrigerator for up to 3 days or in the freezer for up to 1 month.

VARIANT: Dark Chocolate Pinwheels

These pinwheels are decadent and exquisitely balanced between sweet and bitter for a perfect dessert experience. If the Signature Cinnamon Scrolls aren't your favorite, it's probably because these are.

SKILL LEVEL: INTERMEDIATE
COLOR: YELLOW/BROWN
KEYWORDS: SWEET, RICH, VEGETARIAN

Makes 12 large rolls

DOUGH
Same as Signature Cinnamon
    Scrolls

FILLING
½ cup brown sugar, plus more for
    the bottom of the baking pan
5 tablespoons unsalted butter,
    softened, plus 1 tablespoon,
    melted, for brushing

1 cup dark chocolate chips
Pinch of grated nutmeg
Vanilla Cream Cheese Buttercream
    Frosting (page 169)

EQUIPMENT
Same as Signature Cinnamon
    Scrolls, plus:
    Food processor

Step 1: Add the warm milk, warm water, and honey to the bowl of a stand mixer. Sprinkle the yeast on top and allow to bloom for 5 minutes, until frothy.

Step 2: Add the egg, salt, and orange juice to the bowl and combine using a dough hook. Set it to Stir or the lowest setting. Add 2 cups of the flour and allow it to incorporate for 2 to 3 minutes.

Step 3: Make a tangzhong roux (see page 14) using the ⅓ cup milk and ¼ cup of the flour. Add the roux to the stand mixer and increase the speed of the mixer to 3 or Medium-Low. Add the remaining flour in ½-cup increments, allowing the flour to fully incorporate. Stop adding flour when the dough starts to pull a little from the sides of the bowl. Knead for 7 to 9 minutes. The dough should be smooth and elastic, and slightly sticky to the touch.

Step 4: Spray a large bowl with cooking spray. Put the dough into the bowl, cover with a kitchen towel, and allow it to rise in a warm, draft-free place for 1½ to 2 hours, until doubled in bulk.

Step 5: Punch down the dough and roll the dough out with a floured rolling pin on a lightly floured surface into a rectangle about the size of a 13 × 9-inch baking pan.

Step 6: Make the filling: Combine the brown sugar, butter, dark chocolate chips, and nutmeg in the bowl of a food processor. Coarsely mix them together.

Step 7: Spread the mixture onto the rolled-out dough. Press the mixture into the dough with a fork. Roll the dough along the long side into a log, pressing down lightly as you go, pinching the dough sealed.

Step 8: Put the parchment paper into the bottom of a 13 × 9-inch baking pan. Spray it with cooking spray and sprinkle a bit of brown sugar on the parchment paper. Cut the dough into 14 evenly sized sections, discarding the end pieces. Place the rolls in the pan, a few inches apart.

Step 9: Cover the pan with a kitchen towel and allow to rise in a warm, draft-free place for 30 minutes, or until doubled in bulk. RECIPE CONTINUES

Step 10: Preheat the oven to 350°F. Brush the tops of the rolls with the melted butter and place on the middle rack of the oven. Bake for 15 minutes. Rotate the pan to allow it to bake evenly and bake for another 15 minutes, or until golden brown and delicious.

Step 11: Remove the dark chocolate swirls from the oven and allow to cool to room temperature before frosting. Leftovers will keep, tightly covered in the pan, in the refrigerator for up to 3 days or in the freezer for up to 1 month.

Vanilla Cream Cheese Buttercream Frosting

With an equal measure of butter and cream cheese, this frosting floats in homeostasis as neither too sweet nor too tangy. I've had requests for just buckets of this frosting as dessert, to be consumed with a spoon.

SKILL LEVEL: EASY

COLOR: WHITE

KEYWORDS: CREAMY, SWEET, TANGY, VEGETARIAN

Makes 2 cups frosting (enough for a 13 × 9-inch baking pan)

4 tablespoons (½ stick) unsalted butter, at room temperature

4 tablespoons cream cheese, at room temperature

1½ teaspoons vanilla extract

Pinch of kosher salt

2 cups confectioners' sugar

1 to 2 tablespoons heavy cream (optional)

EQUIPMENT

Stand mixer with the paddle attachment

Measuring spoons

Measuring cups

Offset spatula, for frosting

STEP 1: Place the butter and cream cheese in the bowl of a stand mixer and cream together with the speed on Stir. Increase the speed to 3 and add the vanilla and salt.

STEP 2: Slowly add the confectioners' sugar until fully incorporated. Increase the speed one level at a time and beat until fluffy. If more creaminess is desired, add a bit of heavy cream.

STEP 3: Frost the Signature Cinnamon Scrolls, Dark Chocolate Pinwheels, a cake, or a spoon.

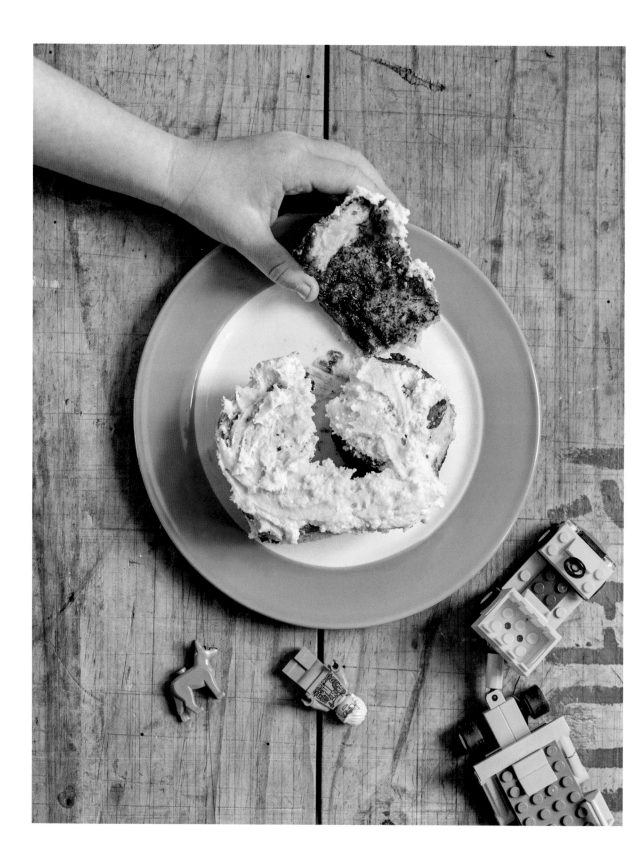

VARIANT: Double Dark Chocolate Cream Cheese Buttercream Frosting

INGREDIENTS

Same as above, plus:

⅓ cup dark or Dutch-process cocoa powder

2 ounces dark chocolate, chopped

EQUIPMENT

Double boiler or microwave-safe bowl

Mixing spoon or spatula

Step 1: Place the butter and cream cheese in the bowl of a stand mixer and cream together with the speed on Stir. Increase the speed to 3 and add the cocoa powder, vanilla, and salt.

Step 2: Slowly add the confectioners' sugar until fully incorporated. Increase the speed one level at a time and beat until fluffy. If more creaminess is desired, add a bit of heavy cream.

Step 3: Melt all the chopped chocolate almost all the way through, either using a double boiler over low heat and frequently stirring or placing the chopped chocolate in a microwave-safe bowl in a microwave and melting it in 10- to 12-second bursts at 50% to 60% cook power, while stirring between blasts with a mixing spoon or spatula. The chocolate should be almost entirely melted, except for a few solid holdouts—if it's too hot and completely smooth, it will melt the frosting when you work it through. (It's important not to use chocolate chips for this step because they frequently have additives to prevent caking that keep the chocolate from melting smoothly.)

Step 4: After the butter, cream cheese, vanilla, confectioners' sugar, and cocoa have been fully mixed and are starting to look light and fluffy, scrape quarter portions of the melted chocolate into the stand mixer bowl as it continues to whisk. Incorporate completely before adding more chocolate. When finished, you can add some heavy cream if you desire a thinner consistency.

Berry Swirl Cookies

These cookies utilize two doughs: a soft sugar cookie base and a second berry dough. You roll them together like a pinwheel. It's a fun way to incorporate a desired color through the berry swirl. Frozen berries work beautifully in this recipe.

SKILL LEVEL: INTERMEDIATE

COLOR: WHITE, BLUE (OR RED)

KEYWORDS: SWEET, SOFT, TOUCHING

Makes 24 large cookies

1 cup (2 sticks) unsalted butter, at room temperature

1½ cups sugar

2 teaspoons vanilla extract

2 cups all-purpose flour, plus more for dusting

2 teaspoons baking soda

2 teaspoons baking powder

1 teaspoon kosher salt

½ cup frozen berries

EQUIPMENT

Kitchen knife

Cutting board

Measuring cups

Measuring spoons

Food processor

Whisk

Mixing bowls

Plastic wrap

Parchment paper

Rolling pin

Cookie sheet

Cooling rack

STEP 1: Cut the butter into ¼-inch cubes for easier mixing. For the first dough section, cream 1 stick of the butter and 1 cup of the sugar along with 1 teaspoon of the vanilla in a food processor. In a small bowl, whisk together 1 cup of the flour, 1 teaspoon of the baking soda, 1 teaspoon of the baking powder, and ½ teaspoon of the salt.

STEP 2: Add the flour mixture to the creamed butter, sugar, and vanilla mixture and pulse until it is a smooth and soft dough. Wrap the finished dough in plastic wrap and set aside.

STEP 3: Cream the remaining 1 stick butter, ½ cup sugar, and 1 teaspoon vanilla together along with the frozen berries in the food processor. In a small bowl, whisk together the remaining 1 cup flour, 1 teaspoon baking soda, 1 teaspoon baking powder, and ½ teaspoon salt. Add the dry ingredients to the berry mixture and pulse until smooth. It will be less tight than the first section of dough.

STEP 4: Dust two pieces of parchment paper with flour. Roll out the non-berried cookie dough between the two sheets to a 12 × 16-inch rectangle that's ½ inch thick. Put the rolled dough in the refrigerator to chill for up to 30 minutes to make it a little easier to work with.

STEP 5: Do the same with the berried dough. It may take a little more flour on the parchment paper to make the dough workable than the first portion, and that's okay! When you pull the chilled dough out of the refrigerator, peel the top layer of parchment paper off slowly and stack both portions over each other, then replace the parchment paper on top and roll a little tighter together. Put the sandwiched dough in the fridge for up to 30 minutes.

STEP 6: Peel the top layer of parchment off your sandwiched dough and use the remaining paper to help guide your hands as you shape this into a jelly roll, with the long side of the rectangle facing you. Keep the roll tight and go slowly. I prefer to tuck the roll over itself toward me, using my thumbs to prevent the parchment paper from rolling into the forming log. Once you have the dough into a jelly roll, you might want to put it in the freezer for a few minutes to make it easier to cut.

STEP 7: Preheat the oven to 375°F. Line a cookie sheet with parchment paper. Using a sharp, serrated knife, cut the dough into ½-inch-round even cookies and place on the cookie sheet. The cookies are going to expand, so give some space between them.

RECIPE CONTINUES

STEP 8: Place the cookie sheet in the oven and bake for about 12 minutes. You want to prevent excess color from forming, as the cookies are meant to be soft and pillowy, so be careful not to overbake. Cool on the cookie sheet for 5 minutes before transferring to a cooling rack for at least 15 more minutes before enjoying. Leftovers will keep in an airtight container on the counter for up to 2 days, in the refrigerator for up to 4 days, or in the freezer for up to 1 month.

Double-Chocolate Cake

This is the cake to end all cakes. Even people who don't like chocolate or cake have named this as one of the best things they've ever eaten.

SKILL LEVEL: EASY

COLOR: BROWN

KEYWORDS: SWEET, MOIST

Makes 8 large servings

1 cup buttermilk, or ¾ cup plus 2 tablespoons whole milk plus 2 tablespoons distilled white vinegar

1 cup fresh hot coffee

2 teaspoons vanilla extract

½ cup vegetable oil

1¾ cups all-purpose flour

¾ cup dark or Dutch-process cocoa powder

1 teaspoon kosher salt

1½ teaspoons baking powder

1½ teaspoons baking soda

2 cups sugar

2 large eggs

Double Dark Chocolate Cream Cheese Buttercream Frosting (page 173)

EQUIPMENT

Measuring spoons

Measuring cups

Cooking spray or parchment paper

2 (9-inch-round) cake pans or 1 (13 × 9-inch) baking pan

Coffeepot

Stand mixer with the paddle attachment

Mixing bowls

Whisk

Cooling rack

STEP 0 (OPTIONAL): If making your own buttermilk, place 2 tablespoons distilled white vinegar in a measuring cup and add enough whole milk to make 1 cup. Set aside for 5 minutes.

RECIPE CONTINUES

STEP 1: Preheat the oven to 350°F. Spray two 9-inch-round cake pans or a 13 × 9-inch baking pan with cooking spray or line with parchment paper. Combine the coffee, vanilla, buttermilk, and vegetable oil in the bowl of a stand mixer and set to low speed.

STEP 2: Combine the flour, cocoa powder, salt, baking powder, baking soda, and sugar in a medium mixing bowl and whisk together. With the mixer running, slowly add the dry ingredients to the stand mixer bowl. Once all the dry ingredients are incorporated, add one of the eggs. As soon as the egg is fully combined, add the second egg. When you can no longer see the yolk running through the batter, turn off the mixer—you don't want to overbeat your batter or it won't get as good a rise.

STEP 3: Either split the cake batter into two 9-inch-round pans or pour the entire batter into a 13 × 9-inch baking pan. It will be quite thin, and that's okay! Don't tap the pan or try to settle the batter; just put in the oven and bake for 30 to 35 minutes, until a toothpick inserted in the center of the cake comes out clean. Cool for 10 minutes before turning out onto a cooling rack and allow to cool completely before frosting. Top with Double Dark Chocolate Cream Cheese Buttercream Frosting for a particularly sinful experience. Leftovers can be covered tightly on a cake tray and stored in the refrigerator for up to 3 days or in the freezer for up to 1 month.

Triple-Layer Chocolate Cream Pie

Silky smooth chocolate custard, a semisoft dark ganache over the crispy and flaky piecrust, and a whipped cream topping to set off this decadence. It's not too sweet, and each layer offers something different to the experience.

SKILL LEVEL: INTERMEDIATE

COLOR: BROWN, WHITE

KEYWORDS: SWEET, TOUCHING, CRUNCHY, SMOOTH, COLD OR ROOM-TEMPERATURE, VEGETARIAN

Makes 8 servings

1 Sweet Piecrust (page 91)

½ cup dark or Dutch-process cocoa powder

½ cup plus 1 tablespoon sugar

Pinch of kosher salt

8 ounces dark chocolate

2 tablespoons unsalted butter

¼ cup all-purpose flour

2 cups whole milk

2 teaspoons vanilla extract

1½ cups heavy cream

EQUIPMENT

9-inch pie pan

Parchment paper

Pie weights or 2 pounds of dried beans

Fork

Measuring cups

Mixing bowls

Whisk

Microwave-safe bowl

Medium saucepan

Spatula or mixing spoon

Microwave-safe container (optional)

Small saucepan

Measuring spoons

Medium dish

Plastic wrap

Stand mixer with the whisk attachment or hand beater

Knife, for serving

STEP 1: Preheat the oven to 375°F. With the Sweet Piecrust in a pie pan, lightly press a sheet of parchment paper onto the surface. On top of the

RECIPE CONTINUES

parchment paper, place pie weights or the dried beans and evenly distribute around the piecrust.

STEP 2: Bake the piecrust for 15 minutes. Take out of the oven and carefully remove the parchment paper and whatever you've used to weight down the crust. Take a fork and make several docking marks in the bottom of the piecrust every couple of inches or so. Return the piecrust to the oven and bake, uncovered, for about 15 minutes, until the bottom is golden brown. Allow to fully cool.

STEP 3: Put the cocoa powder, ½ cup of the sugar, and the salt in a medium mixing bowl and whisk them together. Slightly melt 4 ounces of the dark chocolate in a separate microwave-safe bowl in the microwave for 15 seconds and stir. Set these aside.

STEP 4: Put the butter in a medium saucepan over medium-low heat and add the flour, cooking for 4 to 5 minutes and stirring frequently. While doing this, heat the milk either in a microwave-safe container in the microwave for 1 to 2 minutes or in a small saucepan over medium-low heat, until it almost boils. Slowly pour the hot milk, ¼ to ⅓ cup at a time, into the butter-flour mixture, whisking steadily.

STEP 5: Once you've added all the milk, slowly add the mixed dry ingredients while whisking until fully incorporated. Cook, stirring frequently, for 3 to 5 minutes. Add the melted dark chocolate and stir, allowing to cook for another 2 to 3 minutes. Remove from the heat and stir in the vanilla. Place in a medium dish and cover with a piece of plastic wrap pressed gently into the top of the chocolate pie mixture to prevent a skin from forming. Chill for 1 to 2 hours, until it's fully cooled and set. It will have a nice jiggle when wiggled.

STEP 6: In a small saucepan over medium-high heat, bring 1 cup of the heavy cream to just shy of a boil. Chop up the remaining 4 ounces dark chocolate into small pieces and place the chocolate in a medium mixing bowl. Pour the hot heavy cream over the dark chocolate and stir it through until smooth and shiny. Cool in the fridge for 1 hour, before spooning into the baked piecrust and placing the piecrust in the fridge for 1 more hour.

STEP 7: Add the chilled filling to the piecrust on top of the dark chocolate ganache layer and smooth the custard. Place in the freezer for 5 to 10 minutes.

STEP 8: Just before cutting and serving, use a stand mixer with a whisk attachment or a hand beater to beat the remaining ½ cup heavy cream, adding the remaining 1 tablespoon sugar slowly as you beat the cream. When the peaks of the cream stand up on their own without falling, you've reached the desired consistency. Top the pie with the whipped cream. Cut into wedges and enjoy. Leftovers can be covered tightly in the pan and stored in the refrigerator for up to 3 days.

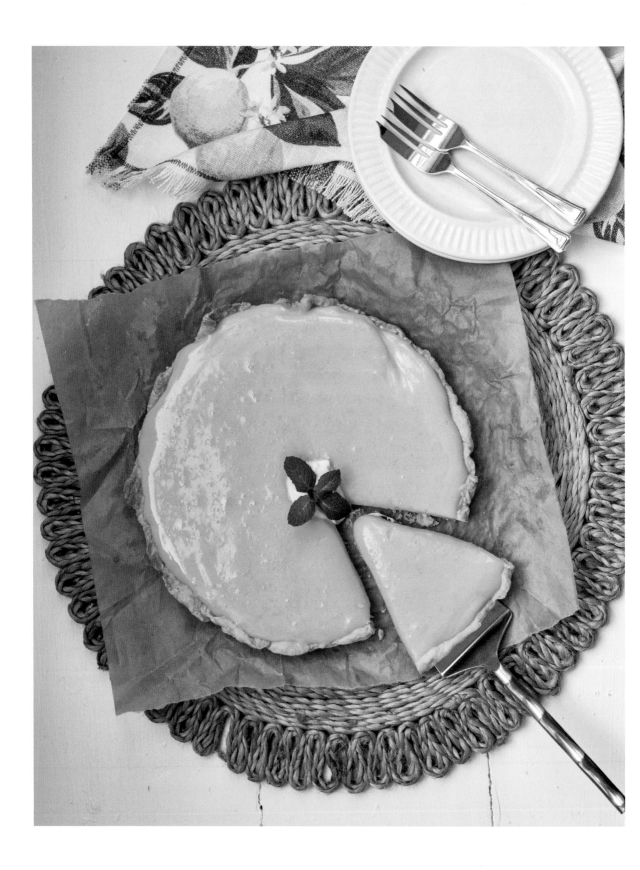

Lemon Tart

There a few things as refreshing as a lemon tart. With a simple sweet piecrust and a tried-and-true lemon curd, you can pull off this dessert that is just out of this world. It's equally balanced between sweet and sour.

SKILL LEVEL: INTERMEDIATE

COLOR: YELLOW

KEYWORDS: SOUR, SWEET, TOUCHING, COLD, GLUTEN-FREE, VEGETARIAN

Makes 8 servings

3 large eggs

¾ cup sugar

Zest of 1 lemon, plus ½ cup fresh lemon juice (1 to 2 large lemons)

Pinch of salt

4 tablespoons (½ stick) cold unsalted butter, cut into cubes

½ teaspoon vanilla extract

1 baked Sweet Piecrust (page 91) (if making for this recipe, add the zest of 1 lemon to the crust)

EQUIPMENT

Medium saucepan

Measuring cups

Microplane or zester

Citrus juicer (optional)

Fork and small mesh strainer (if not using juicer)

Whisk

Wooden spoon

Kitchen knife

Cutting board

Measuring spoons

Storage container

Mixing cups

Plastic wrap

STEP 1: Crack the eggs into a medium saucepan. Add the sugar, lemon zest, lemon juice, and salt. Whisk until the contents are smooth.

STEP 2: Put the saucepan over low heat, while whisking slowly but continuously, mindful to scrape the bottom of the pan. After about 5 minutes, the contents should have thickened considerably. The curd should

RECIPE CONTINUES

coat the back of a wooden spoon, and when you run your finger through the curd on the back of the spoon, the "dammed curd" should retain structural integrity and not immediately rush to fill the space back in.

STEP 3: Remove the saucepan from the heat and gently stir the butter into the warm curd. Once fully incorporated, stir the vanilla into the curd as well. Spoon the contents into a storage container, or keep it in the saucepan during the cooling process. Press some plastic wrap over the curd so that it just touches the surface of the curd, to prevent a skin from developing. Place in the refrigerator for 3 to 4 hours, until fully cooled and set. Will jiggle when wiggled.

STEP 4: Spoon the lemon curd into the prebaked and cooled piecrust. Put it in the freezer for 15 to 20 minutes before cutting and serving. Leftovers can be tightly covered in their pan and stored in the refrigerator for up to 3 days.

ACKNOWLEDGMENTS

This book couldn't have come into this world without a bunch of very special people. First, I'd like to give thanks to Heather Cashman, my nonfiction literary agent, and the team at Storm Literary Agency, who have been my shepherds through this process and to whom I owe a thousand pardons for my manner and ways. My editors with Avery Books, Nina Shield and Hannah Steigmeyer, especially Nina, who had to deal with wrangling me during a pandemic across two continents and hemispheres while with child. Lorie Pagnozzi, the designer, who had an enthusiasm for my project that reinforced how important it is that folks with food aversions are finally getting a cookbook by and for them. And to the countless people I didn't meet at Penguin Random House, yet who played a role in the birth of this book and helped polish it into the gem that it is.

To Charlotte Anderson and Natalie McKenzie, my photographer and food stylist, who welcomed me into their respective families and brought my vision into focus, you're both superstars and this book wouldn't be the same without your touch and the lovely faces of your children enjoying my food.

To the people of New Zealand and Hawke's Bay, especially, who showed only enthusiasm and interest when the odd kilt-wearing American would saunter into their stores to buy ingredients or search for inspiration. Thank you for never making me feel like a stranger.

To Bella, who was hope to me when I never thought I'd see the light of day, I owe the world.

To Finnian, Hunter, Summer, Emma, Joseph, and Freya: You all rock!

To Ewan, my son, I'm sorry I wasn't more patient about the watermelon.

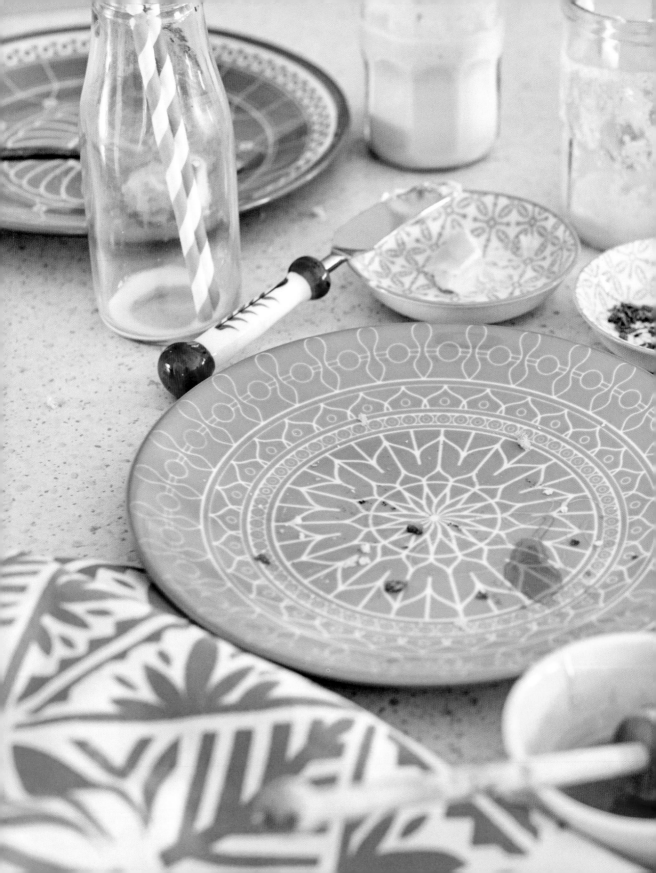

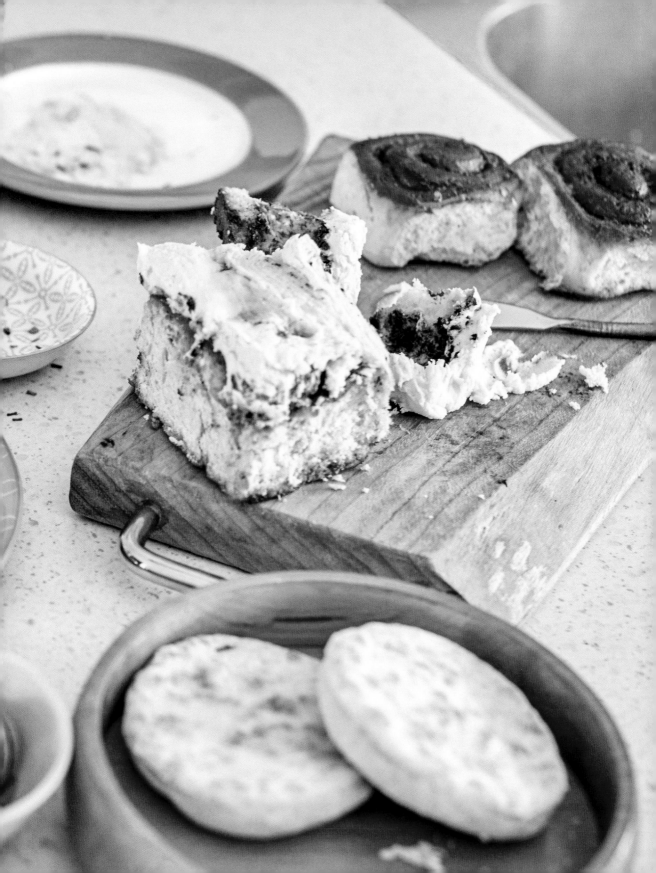

INDEX

Note: Page numbers in *italics* indicate photos.

O

orange (color), aversions/attractions
  about, 24–25
  dinner recipe, 160–61
  lunchtime recipes, 94–96, 120–21

P

pancakes, buttermilk, 74–76
Pan-Fried Salmon Fritters, 151–53
parsnips
  Root Veggie Potpie Filling, 94–96
  Vegan Stuffed Focaccia, 144–45
pasta
  Deconstructed Lasagna, 136–37
  Handmade Pasta, 125–29, 126
  Macaroni and Cheese, 106–9, 107
  Traditional Lasagna, 132, 133–37
Perfect Smashed Cheeseburgers, 103–5, 104
pie, triple-layer chocolate cream, 179–81
piecrusts. See also potpies
  Gluten-Free Vegan Piecrust, 92–93
  Savory Piecrust, 90–91
  Sweet Piecrust, 91–92
pinwheels, dark chocolate, 168–70
plating food
  about: importance of, 43–45
  mixed in ingredients and, 46
  resting dishes before, 49
  sauce/condiment aversions and, 47
  temperature aversions and, 47–49
  touching preference, 45–46
potatoes
  Bacon and Cheese Fries, 111–12
  Filthy Loaded Mashed Potatoes, 99–100
  French Fries, 110–12
  Italian Sausage and Potato Soup, 81–83, 82
  Mashed Potatoes, 97–100
  Root Veggie Potpie Filling, 94–96
  Slightly Dirty Mashed Potatoes, 98–99
potpies
  Chicken Potpie Filling, 94, 96
  Gluten-Free Vegan Piecrust, 92–93
  Root Veggie Potpie Filling, 94–96
  Savory Piecrust, 90–91
pregnancy, cravings and adverse food reactions, 7

profile/worksheet, for food preferences, 8–11
pungent smells, mitigating, 41
pungent taste. See spicy/pungent/capsaicin tastes
purple. See indigo/violet

R

red, aversions/attractions
  about, 24
  dinner recipes, 130–31, 133–37, 144–45, 154–59, 160–61
  lunchtime recipe, 120–21
  treat recipe, 174–76
resting dishes before plating, 49
rice, balancing salty, 18
rich food
  lunchtime recipes, 103–5
  treat recipe, 168–70
Root Veggie Potpie Filling, 94–96. See also Gluten-Free Vegan Piecrust; Savory Piecrust
roux, defined, 3. See also tangzhong method

S

safe veggie time savers, 57. See also no heroes in the kitchen
safety, cooking and, 59
salmon fritters, pan-fried, 151–53
salty food
  about: balancing, 17–18; health and, 17; kosher salt, 150; neutralizing sourness, 19; reducing bitter tastes, 16
  breakfast recipe, 67–69, 70
  dinner recipes (See dinner)
  lunchtime recipes, 79–80, 81–83, 90–96, 97–100, 101–2, 103–5, 106–9, 110–12, 119, 120–21
samefoods, 6–7
sandwiches
  Gluten-Free Sandwich Bread, 116–17
  Grilled Cheese, 118, 119
  Perfect Smashed Cheeseburgers, 103–5, 104
  Sandwich Bread, 113–15, 114
  Stuffed Focaccia, 141–45, 143
sauces
  about: aversions and mitigations, 47; five mother sauces, 3
  Béchamel, 133–34

U

V

W

Y

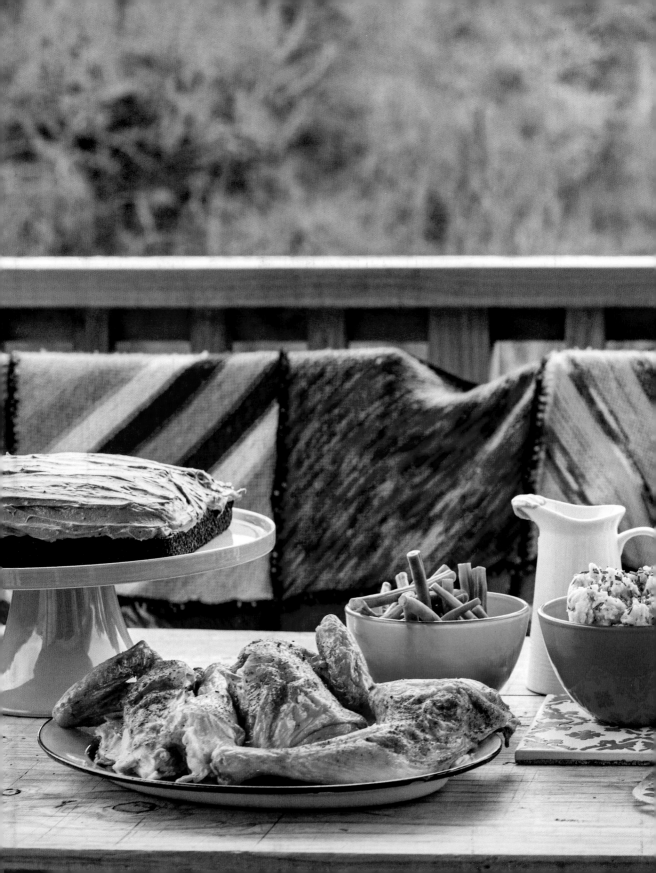